Diagnostic EMQs

Authored by experienced medical professionals, this essential book equips readers with the skills and knowledge needed to excel in the field of medical diagnosis. It is an extensive collection of Extended Matching Questions (EMQs) covering a wide range of topics in general medicine. Each question is accompanied by detailed explanations to provide comprehensive insights. By engaging with these realistic scenarios, readers will develop a deeper understanding of medical conditions, their presentations, and the appropriate diagnostic approaches. The book goes beyond memorization, fostering analytical skills and honing the ability to identify key diagnostic clues within the questions themselves.

KEY FEATURES

- Its comprehensive coverage and focused approach to diagnostic EMQs provide the necessary guidance and practice for medical professionals at multiple levels to excel in assessments and demonstrate proficiency in diagnosing medical conditions. The emphasis on diagnostic approaches and explanations equips readers with the necessary tools to navigate complex scenarios encountered in real-world clinical practice.
- It serves as a much-needed resource for medical professionals preparing for exams, providing a comprehensive collection of diagnostic EMQs not found elsewhere.
- Given the scarcity of available resources specifically tailored to diagnostic EMQs, this book fills a significant gap in the market. Its existence addresses the high demand for comprehensive and targeted study materials for medical examinations. With its focus on enhancing diagnostic reasoning skills, this guide empowers medical professionals to excel in their examinations and effectively diagnose patients, making it an invaluable asset for individuals at various stages of their medical careers. As EMQs are increasingly utilised in medical assessments, having access to a dedicated resource like this becomes crucial for exam preparation.
- By engaging with the extensive collection of diagnostic EMQs in this book, medical professionals can refine their diagnostic reasoning skills and develop a deep understanding of various medical conditions.

MasterPass Series

Spine Surgery Vivas for the FRCS (Tr & Orth)
Kelechi Eseonu, Nicolas Beresford-Cleary

MCQs, MEQs and OSPEs in Occupational Medicine: A Revision Aid
Ken Addley

ENT OSCEs: A guide to your first ENT job and passing the MRCS (ENT) OSCE, 3E
Peter Kullar, Joseph Manjaly, Livy Kenyon

The Final FFICM Structured Oral Examination Study Guide
Eryl Davies

ENT Vivas: A Guide to Passing the Intercollegiate FRCS (ORL–HNS) Viva Examination
Adnan Darr, Karan Jolly, Jameel Muzaffar

Plastic Surgery Vivas for the FRCS (Plast): An Essential Guide
Monica Fawzy

Clinical Consultation Skills in Medicine: A Primer for MRCP PACES
Ernest Suresh

Neurosurgery Second Edition: The Essential Guide to the Oral and Clinical Neurosurgical Exam
Vivian Elwell, Ramez Kirollos, Syed Al-Haddad, Peter Bodkin

Sport and Exercise Medicine: An Essential Guide
David Eastwood, Dane Vishnubala

Refraction and Retinoscopy: How to Pass the Refraction Certificate, Second Edition
Jonathan Park, Leo Feinberg, David Jones

Diagnostic EMQs: A Comprehensive Collection for Medical Examinations
Syed Hussain, Umber Rind, Jawed Noori, Yasmean Kalam, Haseeb Ul Haq Ata, Emmanuel Papageorgiou

For more information about this series please visit: www.routledge.com/MasterPass/book-series/CRCMASPASS

Diagnostic EMQs
A Comprehensive Collection for Medical Examinations

Dr Syed Hussain, BSc, MBBS, FRACGP
Dr Umber Rind, MBBS, FRACGP
Dr Jawed Noori, BMedSci, MBBS, FRACS
Dr Yasmean Kalam, BSc, MBBS
Dr Haseeb Ul Haq Ata, MBBS
Dr Emmanuel Papageorgiou, BMedSsci,
MBBS, FRACGP

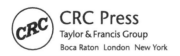

CRC Press
Taylor & Francis Group
Boca Raton London New York

CRC Press is an imprint of the
Taylor & Francis Group, an **informa** business

Cover Image: Shutterstock ID 1714172986

First edition published 2024
by CRC Press
2385 NW Executive Center Drive, Suite 320, Boca Raton FL 33431

and by CRC Press
4 Park Square, Milton Park, Abingdon, Oxon, OX14 4RN

CRC Press is an imprint of Taylor & Francis Group, LLC

© 2024 Syed Hussain, Umber Rind, Jawed Noori, Yasmean Kalam, Haseeb Ul Haq Ata and Emmanuel Papageorgiou

ISBN: 978-1-032-60632-3 (hbk)
ISBN: 978-1-032-60630-9 (pbk)
ISBN: 978-1-003-45994-1 (ebk)

DOI: 10.1201/9781003459941

Typeset in Times
by Apex CoVantage, LLC

For our families—we could not have completed this work without their support. Salma, we will forever miss your encouragement and kind words.

Contents

Acknowledgments   xiii
Author Biographies   xv
Preface   xvii

1 Gastroenterology   **1**
Bowel Conditions 1   1
Bowel Conditions 2   2
Bowel Conditions 3   3
Esophageal Disorders 1   5
Esophageal Disorders 2   6
Gastric Disorders 1   7
Gastric Disorders 2   8
Gastrointestinal Conditions (Paediatric) 1   8
Gastrointestinal Conditions (Paediatric) 2   10
Gastrointestinal Imaging 1   11
Gastrointestinal Imaging 2   11
Gastrointestinal Imaging 3   12
Hepatobiliary Disease 1   13
Hepatobiliary Disease 2   14
Hepatobiliary Disease 3   15
Lumps and Hernias 1   16
Lumps and Hernias 2   17
Perianal Conditions 1   18
Perianal Conditions 2   19
Paediatric Jaundice 1   19
Paediatric Jaundice 2   20
Answers   22

2 Dermatology   **32**
Childhood Infections 1   32
Childhood Infections 2   33
Skin Reactions   34
Hair   35
Nails 1   36
Nails 2   38
Nail Signs of Systemic Illness   39
Dermatitis 1   39

Dermatitis 2   40
Inflammatory Disorders 1   41
Inflammatory Disorders 2   42
Skin Lesions 1   43
Skin Lesions 2   44
Pigmentation Disorders 1   45
Pigmentation Disorders 2   46
Answers   48

3 **Psychiatry**   **55**
Mood Disorders 1   55
Mood Disorders 2   56
Sleep Disturbances 1   57
Sleep Disturbances 2   58
Anxiety 1   59
Anxiety 2   60
Behavioural Conditions 1   61
Behavioural Conditions 2   62
Memory 1   63
Memory 2   65
Paraphilic Conditions 1   66
Paraphilic Conditions 2   67
Personality Disorders 1   68
Personality Disorders 2   69
Substance Related and Addictive Disorders 1   70
Substance Related and Addictive Disorders 2   71
Eating Disorders 1   73
Eating Disorders 2   74
Answers   75

4 **Neurology**   **83**
Cranial Nerve Pathology   83
Dizziness   84
Epilepsy 1   85
Epilepsy 2   86
Facial Pain   88
Headache 1   89
Headache 2   90
Hearing Loss 1   91
Hearing Loss 2   92
Movement Disorders 1   93
Movement Disorders 2   94
Neuromuscular Disorders 1   95
Neuromuscular Disorders 2   97
Vision Loss 1   98
Vision Loss 2   99
Answers   101

5 Women's and Sexual Health   **108**
Amenorrhoea 1   108
Amenorrhoea 2   109
Breast Pathology 1   110
Breast Pathology 2   111
Breast Pathology 3   113
Menstrual Irregularities 1   114
Menstrual Irregularities 2   115
Male Infertility 1   116
Male Infertility 2   117
Complications of Pregnancy 1   118
Complications of Pregnancy 2   119
Vulvovaginal Pathology 1   120
Vulvovaginal Pathology 2   121
Female Infertility 1   122
Female Infertility 2   123
Obstetric Complications 1   124
Obstetric Complications 2   126
Dysmenorrhoea   127
Sexually Transmitted Infection 1   128
Sexually Transmitted Infection 2   129
Genetic Disorders 1   130
Genetic Disorders 2   131
Pelvic-Abdominal Pain 1   132
Pelvic-Abdominal Pain 2   133
Answers   135

6 Urology   **146**
Penis Disorders   146
Testicular and Scrotal Disorders 1   147
Testicular and Scrotal Disorders 2   148
Testicular and Scrotal Disorders 3   150
Urology 1   151
Urology 2   152
Answers   154

7 Musculoskeletal   **158**
Ankle and Shin 1   158
Ankle and Shin 2   159
Back Pain 1   160
Back Pain 2   162
Elbow and Forearm 1   163
Elbow and Forearm 2   164
Foot Pain 1   165
Foot Pain 2   166
Foot Pain 3   167
Hand and Wrist 1   168

Hand and Wrist 2   170
Hip Pain 1   171
Hip Pain 2   172
Knee Pain 1   173
Knee Pain 2   174
Neck and Shoulder Pain 1   176
Neck and Shoulder Pain 2   177
Answers   178

8 **Cardiology**   **187**
Chest Pain 1   187
Chest Pain 2   188
Cardiac Vessels   189
Collapse 1   190
Collapse 2   191
Arrhythmias 1   192
Arrhythmias 2   193
Hypertension 1   194
Hypertension 2   195
Murmurs 1   196
Murmurs 2   197
CHA_2DS_2-VASc Scoring   198
Hypertension Grading   199
Heart Failure Grading   199
Cardiac Structure 1   200
Cardiac Structure 2   201
Answers   203

9 **Respiratory**   **211**
Arterial Blood Gas Interpretation 1   211
Arterial Blood Gas Interpretation 2   212
ENT 1   212
ENT 2   214
Paediatric Respiratory 1   215
Paediatric Respiratory 2   216
Paediatric Respiratory 3   217
Respiratory Conditions 1   218
Respiratory Conditions 2   220
Respiratory Conditions 3   221
Respiratory Conditions 4   222
Pneumothorax   224
Occupational Respiratory Conditions 1   225
Occupational Respiratory Conditions 2   226
Lung Cancer   228
Chest Imaging Findings 1   229

Chest Imaging Findings 2   229
Chest Imaging Findings 3   230
Respiratory Microbiology 1   231
Respiratory Microbiology 2   232
Answers   234

Index   245

Acknowledgments

A special thanks to Dr Ikram Kalam and Dr Syed Murtaza Hussain for their assistance in editing and proofreading the book content. We would also like to acknowledge and thank Rahman Abdul, Shikofa Azizullah, and Reanna Schache for their support and participation in the completion of the book. Finally, thank you Ali and Zain for your patience.

Author Biographies

Syed Hussain brings a wealth of expertise to the book. With extensive experience in emergency medicine and a background that includes a BSc (Botany), MBBS, and FRACGP, his knowledge is invaluable. He has worked in rural regions of Victoria, gaining firsthand understanding of healthcare challenges in diverse settings. Driven by a passion for medical education, he is actively involved in mentoring medical students, particularly in general practice and emergency medicine. With his contributions, *Diagnostic EMQs* becomes an essential resource, providing aspiring medical professionals with the tools to excel in diagnostics and patient care.

Umber Rind is a dedicated medical professional with an MBBS and FRACGP. Her passion lies in women's health and indigenous health. As the owner of a GP clinic, she focuses on providing holistic care to women and indigenous communities. Dr Rind's commitment extends to medical education, where she actively mentors and educates aspiring medical professionals. Her expertise and experiences in these areas enrich the content of the book, making it an invaluable resource for students. Dr Rind's contributions ensure that *Diagnostic EMQs* addresses the unique healthcare needs of these populations, empowering future doctors to deliver quality care.

Jawed Noori is a skilled general surgeon with an impressive academic background. Holding a BMedSci, MBBS, and FRACS, he brings a wealth of knowledge and expertise to the book. With a focus on surgical care, Dr Noori's contributions to the book ensure a comprehensive understanding of surgical conditions and approaches. His extensive experience in the field of general surgery enhances the practicality and relevance of the content. Dr Noori's involvement in *Diagnostic EMQs* strengthens its value as an essential resource for medical students seeking a comprehensive understanding of diagnostic processes in surgical contexts.

Yasmean Kalam is an accomplished medical professional with a diverse academic background. Holding a BSc, MBBS, and currently serving as an anaesthetic fellow, she brings a wealth of expertise to the book. Dr Kalam's contributions focus on anaesthesia, providing essential insights into this critical field. Her comprehensive understanding of anaesthesia, coupled with her commitment to patient care, ensures the practical relevance of the content.

Haseeb Ul Haq Ata is an emergency medicine registrar with extensive experience and a keen interest in trauma management and general emergency medicine. Dr Ata's commitment extends to mentoring aspiring medical professionals, sharing his expertise and experiences. He stays at the forefront of advancements, ensuring the highest standard of care. Dr Ata's passion and dedication empower future doctors to provide quality health-care, making him a valued contributor to this publication.

Emmanuel Papageorgiou is an accomplished medical professional with a BMedSci, MBBS, and FRACGP. He has a special interest in men's health and mental health. His expertise allows him to provide comprehensive care, addressing the unique health-care needs of male patients while ensuring optimal mental wellbeing. Dr Papageorgiou remains up-to-date with the latest research and advancements in his fields of interest. Beyond patient care, he actively contributes to medical education, sharing his knowledge and mentoring aspiring healthcare providers.

Preface

Enhance your diagnostic prowess with *Diagnostic EMQs: A Comprehensive Guide for Medical Examinations*. Authored by experienced medical professionals, this essential book equips you with the skills and knowledge needed to excel in the field of medical diagnosis.

Inside this comprehensive guide, you'll find an extensive collection of extended matching questions (EMQs) covering a wide range of topics in general medicine. These carefully crafted questions challenge your diagnostic reasoning and encourage critical thinking. Each question is accompanied by detailed explanations, drawing upon the authors' clinical expertise to provide comprehensive insights into the diagnostic process.

By engaging with these realistic scenarios, you'll develop a deeper understanding of medical conditions, their presentations, and the appropriate diagnostic approaches. The book goes beyond memorization, fostering analytical skills and honing your ability to identify key diagnostic clues within the questions themselves.

Whether you're a final year medical student or a medical graduate aiming to strengthen your diagnostic abilities, *Diagnostic EMQs* is an indispensable resource. Its structured approach and systematic guidance provide a solid foundation for success in your medical career.

Gastroenterology

1

BOWEL CONDITIONS 1

A. Bowel perforation
B. Carcinoid syndrome
C. Crohn's disease
D. Diverticulitis
E. Irritable bowel syndrome
F. Ischaemic colitis
G. Large bowel obstruction
H. Meckel's diverticulum
I. Ogilvie syndrome
J. Pseudomembranous colitis
K. Short gut syndrome
L. Small bowel obstruction
M. Small intestinal bacterial overgrowth
N. Toxic megacolon
O. Ulcerative colitis

For each of the following, what is the MOST likely diagnosis?

1. A 75-year-old male presents with a six-hour history of colicky lower abdominal discomfort and distension. He tells you that he has not passed wind or opened his bowel for the past 24 hours. On examination he has an empty rectum. You arrange for an erect abdominal X-ray which reveals dilation of the small bowel and colon to the junction of the distal transverse colon and collapse distal to this.

2. A 27-year-old man presents with a six-month history of intermittent abdominal pain associated with diarrhoea. He reports a loss of appetite and a loss of four kg during this time. He has no significant medical history and takes no medication. On examination he has generalised abdominal tenderness but no guarding or rebound tenderness, he also has aphthous ulcers in his mouth. Abdominal X-ray demonstrates a featureless colon. Colonoscopy is arranged and a biopsy is taken which shows a non-caseating granuloma on histology.

3. A 33-year-old male presents with colicky central abdominal pain for the past 12 hours, shortly after it started, he had multiple episodes of bilious

DOI: 10.1201/9781003459941-1

vomiting. He has not opened his bowels since yesterday. He had an appendicectomy at the age of 12 and takes no regular medication. On examination he has a distended abdomen with generalised tenderness and high-pitched bowel sounds. You arrange for an erect abdominal X-ray which reveals distended loops of small bowel with multiple air fluid levels, there is no air seen in the large bowel.

4. A 23-year-old woman presents with a four-month history of almost daily abdominal pain and cramping. Her stool frequency has become irregular and alternates between constipation and diarrhoea. She tells you that her abdominal pain is relieved by defecation. She has no significant medical history and takes a multivitamin daily. On examination she has a mildly distended abdomen but examination is otherwise unremarkable.

5. A 1-year-old boy presents to your emergency department with a two-day history of painless rectal bleeding. His mother reports that the blood is dark red in colour. He has no other symptoms and she reports that he is otherwise well. He has no significant medical history. On examination he has a temperature of 36.5°C, BP of 102/72 mmHg, heart rate of 110 beats per minute and a respiratory rate of 28 breaths per minute. He appears pale, he has a soft and non-tender abdomen. Laboratory investigations reveal microcytic, normochromic anaemia with a haemoglobin of 95 g/L.

See page 22 for answers.

BOWEL CONDITIONS 2

A. Bowel perforation
B. Carcinoid syndrome
C. Crohn's disease
D. Diverticulitis
E. Irritable bowel syndrome
F. Ischaemic colitis
G. Large bowel obstruction
H. Meckel's diverticulum
 I. Ogilvie syndrome
J. Pseudomembranous colitis
K. Short gut syndrome
L. Small bowel obstruction
M. Small intestinal bacterial overgrowth
N. Toxic megacolon
O. Ulcerative colitis

For each of the following, what is the MOST likely diagnosis?

1. A 32-year-old man presents to your clinic complaining of intermittent abdominal cramping associated with watery diarrhoea. He also reports that he has been experiencing facial flushing. Laboratory investigations reveal an elevated urinary 5-hyroxyindoleacetic acid (5-HIAA). An abdominal CT reveals a soft tissue mass lesion in the right iliac fossa and a liver lesion.

2. A 32-year-old woman presents to you with a four-hour history of generalised abdominal pain and swelling. She is three days post-partum and has a healthy child who was delivered via emergency caesarean section after failure to progress in the first stage of labour. She has no significant medical history and takes no medication. On examination she has a markedly distended abdomen with resonance to percussion. Abdominal X-ray reveals significantly dilated loops of large bowel, with a maximal caecal diameter of 12 cm.

3. A 50-year-old woman presents with generalised abdominal pain and fever for the past 24 hours. She has a history of hyperlipidaemia, asthma, and ulcerative colitis. On examination she has a temperature of 38.7°C, tacchycardia, and a distended abdomen with guarding and rebound tenderness throughout. An abdominal X-ray reveals loss of haustra and a significantly distended transverse colon to 9 cm.

4. A 68-year-old male was admitted for repair of an abdominal aortic aneurysm. Shortly after surgery he developed severe generalised abdominal pain associated with bloody diarrhoea. He has a history of T2DM, hypertension, and hypercholesterolaemia. On examination he has a temperature of 37.1 °C, BP 100/72 mmHg, HR 110, SPO2 96% and there is tenderness on the left side of the abdomen. You arrange for a CT of his abdomen which reveals bowel wall thickening and associated fat stranding.

5. A 32-year-old man presents to your ED with acute central abdominal pain. The pain is sharp and severe, it is made worse by movement. The patient has vomited multiple times in your ED with bilious vomits. He has a history of diverticulitis and asthma but takes no regular medication. On examination he has generalised abdominal pain. You arrange an erect abdominal X-ray which demonstrates free air under the diaphragm.

See page 22 for answers.

BOWEL CONDITIONS 3

A. **Bowel perforation**
B. **Carcinoid syndrome**
C. **Crohn's disease**
D. **Diverticulitis**
E. **Irritable bowel syndrome**

F. Ischaemic colitis
G. Large bowel obstruction
H. Meckel's diverticulum
I. Ogilvie syndrome
J. Pseudomembranous colitis
K. Short gut syndrome
L. Small bowel obstruction
M. Small intestinal bacterial overgrowth
N. Toxic megacolon
O. Ulcerative colitis

For each of the following, what is the MOST likely diagnosis?

1. A 26-year-old woman presents to your clinic with a two-year history of abdominal bloating, constipation and flatulence. Over the course of a month you arrange for blood tests, an abdominal ultrasound and an CT abdomen but find no cause behind her symptoms. A glucose hydrogen breath test is arranged which shows a rise in hydrogen.

2. A 68-year-old woman presents with severe diarrhoea for the past four weeks and loss of 8 kg over this period of time. One month prior to her presentation she had surgery for an internal hernia with a large segment of small bowel ischemia.

3. A 63-year-old woman with a BMI of 24 presents with worsening left lower abdominal discomfort. She tells you it started three days ago and has gradually worsened. She has had a hysterectomy and bilateral oophorectomy; she also has a history of hypertension and hyperlipidaemia. On examination she has a temperature of 38.3°C and tenderness in the lower left abdomen and a palpable mass.

4. A 23-year-old woman presents with a two-day history of loose motions associated with mucus initially but now with traces of blood. She has no significant past medical history and takes no regular medication. You arrange for a colonoscopy which demonstrates mucosal inflammation extending from the rectum to 30 cm from the anal verge, there is loss of vascular markings and the mucosa bleeds when touched with the colonoscope, there is normal mucosa beyond this.

5. You are a locum doctor who is called to review a 78-year-old woman at a residential aged care facility. She has had a two-day history of watery diarrhoea. You review her file and note that five days ago she was started on amoxicillin and doxycycline for management of a chest infection.

See page 23 for answers.

ESOPHAGEAL DISORDERS 1

A. Achalasia
B. Barrett esophagus
C. Boerhaave syndrome
D. Diffuse esophageal spasm
E. Eosinophilic esophagitis
F. Esophageal candidiasis
G. Esophageal cancer
H. Esophageal varices
I. Gastroesophageal reflux
J. Mallory–Weiss tear
K. Viral esophagitis
L. Zenker's diverticulum

For each of the following, what is the MOST likely diagnosis?

1. A 27-year-old HIV positive male presents to ED with a three-day history of sore throat, chest discomfort and odynophagia. He has recently been unwell with muscle aches, pains, low grade temperatures and coryzal symptoms. He tells you that he has epigastric and retrosternal pain that radiates through to his back with swallowing. On examination he has pharyngeal and bilateral tonsillar erythema. You arrange for a gastroscopy which reveals four well demarcated ulcers of the esophagus.

2. A 23-year-old university student has been vomiting violently for two hours with streaks of blood in the most recent vomitus. He has been out with friends drinking heavily tonight.

3. A 66-year-old male presents with a six-month history of dysphagia and odynophagia. He explains that when his symptoms first began, he had difficulty swallowing solids but over the past two months he has found difficulty with fluids. During this time, he has lost 15 kg. He has a raspy voice and a BMI of 17.

4. A 56-year-old woman presents with central chest pain and discomfort, she has a long history of reflux and takes esomeprazole daily to help with this. She has a history significant for asthma and scleroderma. You refer her to a gastroenterologist who arranges for a gastroscopy. The mucosa in the lower half of the esophagus demonstrates a red and velvety appearance.

5. A 56-year-old homeless male presents to your emergency department with haematemesis. He has no known past medical history and denies any medication use. Examination reveals palmar erythema, spider naevi, hepatomegaly and caput medusa.

See page 23 for answers.

ESOPHAGEAL DISORDERS 2

A. **Achalasia**
B. **Barrett esophagus**
C. **Boerhaave syndrome**
D. **Diffuse esophageal spasm**
E. **Eosinophilic esophagitis**
F. **Esophageal candidiasis**
G. **Esophageal cancer**
H. **Esophageal varices**
 I. **Gastroesophageal reflux**
J. **Mallory–Weiss tear**
K. **Viral esophagitis**
L. **Zenker's diverticulum**

For each of the following, what is the MOST likely diagnosis?

1. A 48-year-old woman presents with a history of weight loss, she reports that she has dysphagia for both solids and liquids. You arrange for a barium swallow which reveals tapering of the lower esophageal sphincter with narrowing at the gastroesophageal junction producing a rat's tail like appearance.

2. A 24-year-old woman has a six-month history of retrosternal chest pain associated with a sour taste in her mouth. She explains that on occasion she feels symptoms at night when she is lying down and has to adjust her position. Her symptoms occur at least two times a week. She has no loss of weight or appetite.

3. A 21-year-old nursing student presents with a long history of "food getting stuck" in her throat with most meals. She explains that she has had to chew her food for longer periods of time and drink plenty of water to help with passage of each bolus. She has a history of eczema and asthma. You send her for a gastroscopy which reveals a narrowed esophagus with edema, white exudates, trachealisation of the esophagus and longitudinal furrows. Biopsy of esophagus reveals 29 eosinophils per high power field from the distal esophagus.

4. A 53-year-old man complains of a long history of chest pain associated with swallowing, sometimes causing regurgitation of food. He explains that his symptoms are episodic and are worsening with time. You arrange for a barium swallow which reveals a corkscrew esophagus.

5. A 14-year-old boy presents to your clinic complaining of a six-week history of epigastric discomfort and odynophagia. He tells you that his symptoms have been worsening over the past fortnight. He does not have a reduced appetite and has not experienced weight loss during this period of time. He has a history of eczema and asthma. He currently uses Ventolin and was recently commenced on budesonide for worsening asthma symptoms.

See page 24 for answers.

GASTRIC DISORDERS 1

A. Coeliac disease
B. Dumping syndrome
C. Duodenal ulcer
D. Gastric cancer
E. Gastric ulcer
F. Gastroenteritis
G. Gastroparesis
H. Hiatus hernia
I. Perforated peptic ulcer
J. Zollinger–Ellison syndrome

For each of the following, what is the MOST likely diagnosis?

1. A 53-year-old woman presents with a six-month history of epigastric discomfort. She reports that she has had severe nausea, reflux, loss of appetite and has lost 8 kg during this time. She has no significant medical history and takes no regular medication. You arrange for a barium swallow which reveals thickened stiff walls in the stomach creating a leather water bottle appearance.

2. A 42-year-old woman presents with a six-month history of abdominal discomfort, loss of weight and difficulty in flushing stools. You send her for pathology which reveals the presence of anti-gliadin antibodies. She is referred to a gastroenterologist who arranges for endoscopy and duodenal biopsy which reveals intra-epithelial lymphocytosis with blunting of villi.

3. A 54-year-old male presents to your GP clinic complaining of a six-month history of intermittent episodes of sweats, palpitations, lightheadedness and tremors. The episodes last for a few minutes and occur most commonly after high sugar intake. He has a history of hypertension, hyperlipidaemia and diet controlled T2DM. He had a gastric bypass procedure two years ago for weight loss. His current medications are Ramipril and Atorvastatin. On examination he has a RR of 18, BP of 124/66 mmHg, temperature of 36.5°C and has a BMI of 33.

4. A 32-year-old woman presents with a 12-month history of epigastric discomfort, postprandial fullness and intermittent vomiting. She has no significant medical history and uses no regular medications. You arrange for a chest X-ray which reveals retrocardiac opacity with a single air-fluid level.

See page 24 for answers.

GASTRIC DISORDERS 2

A. Coeliac disease
B. Dumping syndrome
C. Duodenal ulcer
D. Gastric cancer
E. Gastric ulcer
F. Gastroenteritis
G. Gastroparesis
H. Hiatus hernia
I. Perforated peptic ulcer
J. Zollinger–Ellison syndrome

For each of the following, what is the MOST likely diagnosis?

1. A 52-year-old male presents with upper abdominal discomfort which he reports is worse at night and relieved with eating. He has been vomiting up small amounts of blood in the past few hours. He has not noticed any bowel changes or blood per rectum, and has not had any loss of weight or loss of appetite.

2. A 56-year-old man presents with epigastric pain that has been ongoing and not improving for the past few days. In the past 24 hours he reports that he has had small amounts of haematemesis. He has a history of lower back pain and osteo-arthritis and takes regular paracetamol and ibuprofen. He tells you that eating food makes his symptoms worse.

3. A 68-year-old male presents with acute onset epigastric discomfort. The pain started 30 minutes ago and is worse with movement and coughing. He has a history of osteoarthritis and hypertension. He currently uses Ramipril daily and has found much relief with ibuprofen which he takes up to four times a day. You arrange for an erect abdominal X-ray which reveals pneumoperitoneum.

4. A 22-year-old nurse presents with a two-day history of loose motions and vomiting. She reports that during this time she has had a headache, sweats, muscle aches and pains. On examination she has a RR of 20, BP of 106/72 mmHg, temperature of 38.1 °C and dry mucous membranes.

See pages 24–25 for answers.

GASTROINTESTINAL CONDITIONS (PAEDIATRIC) 1

A. Appendicitis
B. Duodenal atresia

C. **Gastroenteritis**
D. **Hirschsprung's disease**
E. **Intussusception**
F. **Meconium ileus**
G. **Mesenteric adenitis**
H. **Necrotising enterocolitis**
I. **Pyloric stenosis**
J. **Sigmoid volvulus**
K. **Wilm's tumor**

For each of the following, what is the MOST likely diagnosis?

1. A 6-week-old girl is brought to your clinic by her concerned parents. She has been vomiting for the past two weeks intermittently and over the past 24 hours has been projectile vomiting shortly after each feed. Despite the vomiting she is persistently hungry, her mum has just fed her in the waiting room before entering your consultation room. On examination she has dry mucous membranes and you palpate an olive shaped mass in the epigastrium.

2. A 10-week-old child presents to your ED with a one-day history of fever and vomiting. His mother tells you that he has had dry nappies and has been constipated for the past three days. He has cystic fibrosis and has been following up with a specialist clinic for this. On examination he has a distended abdomen which is resonant to percussion. An abdominal X-ray is performed which reveals distended loops of bowel with a soap bubble appearance.

3. A 5-year-old boy presents with a three-day history of loose motions and vomiting. His mother explains that he has had sweats, muscle aches and pains. On examination he has a RR of 20, BP of 106/72 mmHg, temperature of 38.1 °C and dry mucous membranes.

4. A 2-year-old child presents to your ED with acute onset of central abdominal discomfort and vomiting associated with red currant jelly stools. He has had intermittent abdominal discomfort over the past two weeks. You palpate his abdomen and note a sausage shaped mass in the central abdomen.

5. A 6-year-old boy presents to your GP clinic with a two-day history of central abdominal pain radiating to the right lower quadrant. On examination he has a RR of 18, BP of 122/84 mmHg, HR 120, temperature of 38.1oC, a tender abdomen with right lower quadrant peritonism and a positive psoas sign.

6. A 3-year-old boy presents to your clinic with his father who has noticed left sided abdominal swelling. On examination there is a palpable mass in the left flank. Urine dipstick reveals haematuria.

See page 25 for answers.

GASTROINTESTINAL CONDITIONS (PAEDIATRIC) 2

A. **Appendicitis**
B. **Duodenal atresia**
C. **Gastroenteritis**
D. **Hirschsprung's disease**
E. **Intussusception**
F. **Meconium ileus**
G. **Mesenteric adenitis**
H. **Necrotising enterocolitis**
I. **Pyloric stenosis**
J. **Sigmoid volvulus**
K. **Wilm's tumor**

For each of the following, what is the MOST likely diagnosis?

1. A 3-day-old attends with his mother who is concerned that he has not had a bowel motion since birth. He has also had bilious vomiting and a distended abdomen. You examine the child and note that he has abdominal distension, flat facial features, small head, short neck and upward slanting eyes, otherwise he examines well. Abdominal X-ray reveals distended loops of bowel down to the descending colon.

2. A 12-year-old boy presents with three-day history of generalised colicky abdominal pain which started on the left side, it is associated with vomiting, constipation and nausea. On examination he has an asymmetrically distended abdomen with exaggerated bowel sounds. Digital rectal examination reveals an empty rectum. You arrange for an abdominal X-ray which reveals dilated sigmoid loop with a coffee bean appearance.

3. A 7-year-old boy presents with a one-day history of worsening umbilical pain. He has recently had a low-grade fever, sore throat and runny nose which are starting to settle. He reports that the pain has moved to the right lower quadrant of the abdomen in the past few hours. On examination he has a RR of 18, BP of 126/78 mmHg, temperature of 37.1°C, and a soft and a negative jump test.

4. A 12-day-old child presents with a distended abdomen, bilious vomiting and decreased urine output. Her symptoms started yesterday. She was born at 29 weeks' gestation and had to spend time in ICU for respiratory distress syndrome. On examination she has a distended abdomen. You arrange an abdominal X-ray which reveals pneumatosis intestinalis.

5. A newborn child with Down syndrome presents with a several hour history of bilious vomiting. You arrange for an abdominal X-ray which reveals a "double bubble" appearance. During her pregnancy the mother reports she had polyhydramnios.

See pages 25–26 for answers.

GASTROINTESTINAL IMAGING 1

A. Achalasia
B. Colorectal carcinoma
C. Crohn's disease
D. Diaphragmatic rupture
E. Diffuse esophageal spasm
F. Duodenal atresia
G. Impending abdominal aortic aneurysm rupture
H. Intraluminal duodenal diverticulum
I. Intussusception
J. Pneumoperitoneum
K. Pyloric stenosis
L. Sigmoid volvulus
M. Small bowel haematoma
N. Small bowel obstruction
O. Ulcerative colitis

For each of the following, what is the MOST likely diagnosis?

1. High attenuating crescent sign seen on CT of the abdomen.
2. Caterpillar sign seen on abdominal X-ray.
3. Double bubble sign seen on abdominal X-ray.
4. Apple core sign seen on barium enema.
5. String of pearls sign seen on erect abdominal X-ray.

See page 26 for answers.

GASTROINTESTINAL IMAGING 2

A. Achalasia
B. Colorectal carcinoma
C. Crohn's disease
D. Diaphragmatic rupture
E. Diffuse esophageal spasm
F. Duodenal atresia
G. Impending abdominal aortic aneurysm rupture
H. Intraluminal duodenal diverticulum
I. Intussusception
J. Pneumoperitoneum
K. Pyloric stenosis
L. Sigmoid volvulus

M. **Small bowel haematoma**
N. **Small bowel obstruction**
O. **Ulcerative colitis**

For each of the following, what is the MOST likely diagnosis?

1. Bird's beak sign seen on barium swallow.
2. Coffee bean sign seen on abdominal X-ray.
3. Cottage loaf sign seen on CT of the abdomen.
4. Target sign seen on abdominal ultrasound.
5. Lead pipe sign seen on an erect abdominal X-ray.

See pages 26–27 for answers.

GASTROINTESTINAL IMAGING 3

A. **Achalasia**
B. **Colorectal carcinoma**
C. **Crohn's disease**
D. **Diaphragmatic rupture**
E. **Diffuse esophageal spasm**
F. **Duodenal atresia**
G. **Impending abdominal aortic aneurysm rupture**
H. **Intraluminal duodenal diverticulum**
I. **Intussusception**
J. **Pneumoperitoneum**
K. **Pyloric stenosis**
L. **Sigmoid volvulus**
M. **Small bowel haematoma**
N. **Small bowel obstruction**
O. **Ulcerative colitis**

For each of the following, what is the MOST likely diagnosis?

1. Stack of coins sign seen on erect abdominal X-ray.
2. Telltale triangle sign seen on plain abdominal X-ray.
3. Corkscrew appearance seen on barium swallow.
4. Ram's horn sign seen on a barium meal.

See page 27 for answers.

HEPATOBILIARY DISEASE 1

A. Alcoholic hepatitis
B. Ascending cholangitis
C. Cholecystitis
D. Choledocholithiasis
E. Dubin–Johnson syndrome
F. Gaucher's disease
G. Gilbert's syndrome
H. Haemochromatosis
I. Hepatitis A
J. Hepatitis B–acute
K. Hepatitis B–chronic
L. Hepatitis B resolved
M. Pancreatic cancer
N. Pancreatitis
O. Primary biliary cirrhosis
P. Primary sclerosing cholangitis
Q. Rotor disease
R. Wilson's disease

For each of the following, what is the MOST likely diagnosis?

1. A 39-year-old man presents with a one-day history of right upper quadrant pain. On examination he has a temperature of 38.1°C and he has a positive Murphy's sign.

2. A 61-year-old male presents with a two-day history of skin colour changes and itch. He has a history of gall stones. On examination he is afebrile, his observations are within a normal range and he is jaundiced. Abdominal examination is unremarkable. ERCP reveals a filling defect in the common bile duct.

3. A 62-year-old male attends your clinic for results of his blood tests, he is asymptomatic today. He has no significant medical history and takes no medication. He migrated from Egypt when he was 21 years of age and lives with his wife and two daughters. He has a raised ALT and AST but the remainder of his bloods are normal. You arrange for follow up bloods which reveal HBsAg positive, anti-HBc positive, IgM anti-HBc negative and anti-HBs negative.

4. A 68-year-old man presents with a two-week history of generalised itch, choluria and skin discoloration. On questioning he explains that he has lost 10 kg in the past six months and has a loss of appetite. On examination he is jaundiced and you palpate a mass in the epigastric region 2 cm below the left costal margin.

5. A 32-year-old hairdresser attends your clinic complaining of fatigue. She tells you that over the past week she has also been nauseated and has had upper abdominal pain. On examination she has normal observations but she is jaundiced and has mild discomfort with palpation of the right upper quadrant. You arrange for

serology which reveals AST 2234, ALT 2006, ALP 122, Bilirubin 24, HBsAg positive, anti-HBc positive, IgM anti-HBc positive and anti-HBs negative.

See page 27 for answers.

HEPATOBILIARY DISEASE 2

A. **Alcoholic hepatitis**
B. **Ascending cholangitis**
C. **Cholecystitis**
D. **Choledocholithiasis**
E. **Dubin–Johnson syndrome**
F. **Gaucher's disease**
G. **Gilbert's syndrome**
H. **Haemochromatosis**
I. **Hepatitis A**
J. **Hepatitis B–acute**
K. **Hepatitis B–chronic**
L. **Hepatitis B–resolved**
M. **Pancreatic cancer**
N. **Pancreatitis**
O. **Primary biliary cirrhosis**
P. **Primary sclerosing cholangitis**
Q. **Rotor disease**
R. **Wilson's disease**

For each of the following, what is the MOST likely diagnosis?

1. A 21-year-old presents with a two-day history of fever and nausea. He tells you that he has also had abdominal cramping and dark urine. He recently returned from Thailand two weeks ago where he had been on a field trip with university visiting various agricultural sites. On examination he has a temperature of 37.9°C, he appears jaundiced, has hepatosplenomegaly and cervical lymphadenopathy.

2. A 45-year-old presents with a one-week history of abdominal swelling and generalised itch. He has a history of hypertension and uses Captopril to treat this. He is a non-smoker and drinks eight cans of full-strength beer on most nights, he has done this for the last 10 years. On examination he appears jaundiced, has decreased chest hair, bilateral gynaecomastia, abdominal distension, multiple spider naevi and hepatomegaly. His abdomen is non tender on palpation. You arrange for bloods which reveal AST 153, ALT 68, ALP 197 and Bilirubin 120.

3. A 37-year-old male presents to your GP clinic. He explains that he has been putting off review with you as he has a phobia of doctor's clinics. He explains that he was meant to come and see a GP many years ago as there is a family history

of liver problems and as a young child he was admitted to hospital because he was jaundiced. You arrange for some blood tests which reveal normal LFT's, HBsAg negative, anti-HBc positive and anti-HBs positive.

4. A 43-year-old woman presents to your emergency department with worsening epigastric pain. She reports that her pain started two hours ago and is severe in nature, radiating through to her back. She gets some relief with leaning forward. She has vomited three times as a result of her symptoms. She has a history of gallstones and takes no regular medication. On examination she is afebrile, observations are within normal limits and she is very tender in the epigastric region. Serology reveals a lipase of 312 U/L.

See pages 27–28 for answers.

HEPATOBILIARY DISEASE 3

A. Alcoholic hepatitis
B. Ascending cholangitis
C. Cholecystitis
D. Choledocholithiasis
E. Dubin–Johnson syndrome
F. Gaucher's disease
G. Gilbert's syndrome
H. Haemochromatosis
 I. Hepatitis A
 J. Hepatitis B – acute
K. Hepatitis B – chronic
L. Hepatitis B – resolved
M. Pancreatic cancer
N. Pancreatitis
O. Primary biliary cirrhosis
P. Primary sclerosing cholangitis
Q. Rotor disease
R. Wilson's disease

For each of the following, what is the MOST likely diagnosis?

1. A 54-year-old woman presents with a long history of fatigue, joint pain, generalised itch and unexplained bruising. She has a history of osteoporosis and hypertension. On examination she has xanthelasma and hepatomegaly. Anti-mitochondrial antibodies are positive.

2. A 38-year-old male presents with fatigue, pruritus and jaundice. He drinks two to three cans of beer a day on weekends and is a non-smoker. He has a history of ulcerative colitis. On examination he is jaundiced and has hepatomegaly. You

arrange for bloods which reveal a significantly elevated ALP. After specialist referral an ERCP is performed which reveals beading of the bile ducts within the liver.

3. A 22-year-old woman presents with recurrent episodes of jaundice for the past three years. Episodes are usually preceded by upper respiratory tract infections. She presents today with mild jaundice. You arrange for liver function tests which reveal normal liver function but a raised bilirubin level.

4. A 56-year-old woman presents with chronic arthralgia and fatigue. She tells you that the pain mostly affects her hands and particularly the 2nd and 3rd MCP joints. Recently she has also noticed abdominal discomfort in the right upper quadrant. On examination you note swelling in all joints of both hands, abdominal exam reveals hepatomegaly. You arrange for serology which reveals serum ferritin of 520 µg/L, transferrin saturation 61%.

5. A 52-year-old male presents with a one-day history of abdominal pain and jaundice. He explains that the pain is severe, in the right upper quadrant and radiating to the right shoulder tip. He reports dark urine and light-coloured stools. On examination he is jaundiced, has a temperature of 38.6°C and Murphy's sign is negative.

See page 28 for answers.

LUMPS AND HERNIAS 1

A. **Direct inguinal hernia**
B. **Divarication of recti**
C. **Epigastric hernia**
D. **Femoral hernia**
E. **Indirect inguinal hernia**
F. **Paraumbilical hernia**
G. **Richter's hernia**
H. **Saphena varix**
 I. **Spigelian hernia**
J. **Umbilical hernia**

For each of the following, what is the MOST likely diagnosis?

1. A 32-year-old multiparous woman presents for her six-week check. She delivered her daughter at term via caesarean section due to breech position. She complains of abdominal muscle weakness. On examination the upper midline bulges when intra-abdominal pressure is increased.

2. A 2-month-old child attends your clinic for the first time with his mother for a routine check-up. On examination you note a bulge in the belly button area. His mother tells you she noticed it a few weeks ago and explains that it swells when he cries or tries to pass a motion.

3. A 36-year-old male presents with a four-month history of pain around his belly button. He tells you he has had a lump there since he was 10 years old and it was pea sized back then. He tells you that four months ago the lump increased to the size of a walnut all of a sudden which was quite painful at the time. It gets larger with Valsalva manoeuvre and reduces with lying down.
4. A 23-year-old tradesman presents with a two-year history of left groin lump. You reduce the lump then apply pressure over the inguinal canal, the patient is asked to cough which causes a bulge against your hand.

See pages 28–29 for answers.

LUMPS AND HERNIAS 2

A. Direct inguinal hernia
B. Divarication of recti
C. Epigastric hernia
D. Femoral hernia
E. Indirect inguinal hernia
F. Paraumbilical hernia
G. Richter's hernia
H. Saphena varix
I. Spigelian hernia
J. Umbilical hernia

For each of the following, what is the MOST likely diagnosis?

1. A 26-year-old woman presents to your clinic complaining of a painless lump in her upper abdomen. She has a past history of endometriosis diagnosed by laparoscopy. On examination you note a small lump measuring 1.5 cm in diameter in the midline between her belly button and her sternum.
2. A 38-year-old man presents to your clinic concerned about a blue tinged lump in his left groin. He has a history of varicose veins, asthma and uses Ventolin on occasion. On examination there is a blue tinged, non-tender, fluctuant soft lump in his left groin which displays a cough impulse. The lump disappears on lying flat.
3. A 38-year-old plumber complains of a one-year history of a lump in his right groin. You reduce the lump then apply pressure over the deep inguinal ring, the patient is asked to cough and you feel it protrude despite occlusion.
4. A 53-year-old primary school teacher presents to your clinic with a lump in her right groin which is not reducible. The lump is below and lateral to the pubic tubercle.

See page 29 for answers.

PERIANAL CONDITIONS 1

A. Anal fissure
B. Condyloma
C. Internal haemorrhoid
D. Molluscum contagiosum
E. Perianal abscess
F. Perianal haematoma
G. Pilonidal sinus
H. Proctalgia fugax
 I. Rectal prolapse
J. Rectal varices
K. Solitary rectal ulcer syndrome

For each of the following, what is the MOST likely diagnosis?

1. A 24-year-old student presents complaining of a one-month history of inter-mittent tight cramping pain around the rectum above his anus. Episodes last for about two minutes and spontaneously resolve. He tells you that they occur mostly at night and cause him to wake up. On examination his abdomen is soft and non-tender, a rectal examination is unremarkable.

2. A 32-year-old hairdresser attends your GP clinic with a complaint of anal itch, he reports that on occasion he notices a small amount of PR bleeding on wiping after defecation. He has had at least three male partners in the past six months. On examination you find small pinhead sized growths on the anal verge.

3. A 33-year-old woman presents with a five-day history of painless rectal bleed-ing. She describes the blood as bright in colour and occurring after defecation. She explains that she notices the blood as being separate from the stools and dripping onto the toilet bowl. No masses protrude from the anus.

4. A 23-year-old university student presents with a two-year history of pain in his lower back associated with intermittent discharge. On examination you note a scar measuring 3 cm with multiple openings on either end in the middle of the natal cleft about 5 cm from the anal verge.

5. A 26-year-old woman presents with a two-day history of excruciating anal pain on defecation associated with haematochezia. The pain lasts for some time after defecation, she also reports that she has been constipated for the past week. She has no significant medical history. You gently perform an anal examination which reveals defect in the skin of the anal canal distal to the dentate line.

6. A 58-year-old obstetrician attends your emergency department complaining of rectal discomfort. She tells you that she has had some PR bleeding over the past 24 hours after an episode of straining while trying to pass a motion. She tells you that she has had constipation for the past few days. On examination you note a rectal mass which gets larger when you ask the patient to perform a Valsalva manoeuvre.

See pages 29–30 for answers.

PERIANAL CONDITIONS 2

A. Anal fissure
B. Condyloma
C. Internal haemorrhoid
D. Molluscum contagiosum
E. Perianal abscess
F. Perianal haematoma
G. Pilonidal sinus
H. Proctalgia fugax
 I. Rectal prolapse
J. Rectal varices
K. Solitary rectal ulcer syndrome

For each of the following, what is the MOST likely diagnosis?

1. A 36-year-old woman presents with a three-month history of rectal pain. On examination you note small flesh-coloured bumps around her anus and vulva which are round and dimpled in their centres.
2. A 62-year-old male presents with a two-day history of inability to defecate due to extreme rectal pain. On examination you observe a dark bluish lump at the verge of the anal canal.
3. A 54-year-old male presents with a two-month history of rectal bleeding associated with abdominal swelling. He tells you that the blood is bright coloured and not associated with pain. He has a history of alcoholism. On examination he has jaundice, hepatomegaly and ascites.
4. A 58-year-old man presents to your GP clinic with rectal pain associated with bleeding, He explains that he has had constipation for the past six months and had been passaging large amounts of mucus with stools. You arrange for colonoscopy which reveals a large ulcer at the 6 cm distance from the anal verge.
5. A 36-year-old reports that he has noticed anal pain for the past two days, he explains that it feels like a throbbing sensation. He tells you that he has also had intermittent sweats and shakes. He tells you his symptoms are worse at the end of the day when he has to sit on the seat of his Vespa. On examination you note a red lump under the skin near the anus which is pea sized and very tender to touch.

See page 30 for answers.

PAEDIATRIC JAUNDICE 1

A. ABO incompatibility
B. Biliary atresia

C. **Breast milk jaundice**
D. **Cephalohaematoma**
E. **Choledochal cyst**
F. **Crigler–Najjar syndrome type 1**
G. **Crigler–Najjar syndrome type 2**
H. **Cystic fibrosis**
I. **Galactosaemia**
J. **G6PD Deficiency**
K. **Hypothyroidism**
L. **Physiological jaundice**
M. **Rhesus incompatibility**

For each of the following, what is the MOST likely diagnosis?

1. A 5-day-old child presents with his mother who is concerned about discoloration in his skin which she noticed two days ago. He was born at term via forceps delivery due to prolonged labour. On examination you note that the child is mildly jaundiced with a large lump at the top of his head.

2. A 2-week-old child attends your emergency department with her concerned parents. She is breastfed, has been vomiting after most feeds, has had ongoing diarrhoea and as a result of her symptoms she has not been thriving. Today her mother explains that she has noticed yellow discoloration of her skin and that she has been very irritable. She was born at home at 39 weeks' gestation via uncomplicated vaginal delivery. Her parents have not registered her birth with local authorities as yet and she has not been seen by a doctor or nurse. On examination she has hepatomegaly and obvious jaundice.

3. A 3-day-old child presents to your clinic with his mother who is concerned about a slight yellow discoloration in his skin which she noticed last night. He is bottle fed and has been feeding well, has normal stools and is passing urine without concern. He was born at term via vaginal delivery without any complications and has no significant family history. On examination his observations are within normal limits.

4. A female infant is born at 38 weeks via vaginal delivery with a birth weight of 2.9 kg to an otherwise healthy 33-year-old mother. Twelve hours after delivery she developed jaundice; she was subsequently admitted. You arrange for bloods which reveal indirect bilirubinaemia and metabolic acidosis. Her parents are both rhesus negative.

See page 30 for answers.

PAEDIATRIC JAUNDICE 2

A. **ABO incompatibility**
B. **Biliary atresia**

C. **Breast milk jaundice**
D. **Cephalohaematoma**
E. **Choledochal cyst**
F. **Crigler–Najjar syndrome type 1**
G. **Crigler–Najjar syndrome type 2**
H. **Cystic fibrosis**
 I. **Galactosaemia**
J. **G6PD Deficiency**
K. **Hypothyroidism**
L. **Physiological jaundice**
M. **Rhesus incompatibility**

For each of the following, what is the MOST likely diagnosis?

1. A 1-month-old child presents with a history of jaundice since the fifth day of life. The child has been passing normal coloured stools and urine. Her mother explains that she has had constipation and has been sleeping excessively. On examination you note a puffy face, prominent tongue and dry skin.
2. A 2-month-old child presents with worsening jaundice. His parents report that he has had yellow discoloration and pale stools over the past four weeks, they did not think much of it. The parents attended their local GP clinic for routine vaccinations and the duty nurse has asked them to attend the ED as she is concerned. On examination he is jaundiced, and has marked hepatomegaly. You arrange for bloods which reveal a raised direct bilirubin, raised transaminases, raised ALP and raised GGT. Ultrasound reveals a positive triangular cord sign and a gall bladder length of 18 mm.
3. A 3-day-old child is brought into your clinic by his mother who is concerned as his skin has changed colour. He was born at term via normal vaginal delivery and is exclusively breastfed. You refer him to your local paediatric unit where his jaundice peaked at day five and then completely resolved by day 12. A discharge summary reveals that when he presented, he had normal LFT's and indirect bilirubinaemia.
4. A 2-year-old child presents to your clinic with a one-day history of jaundice, he has also been passing orange coloured urine. His mother has been introducing new foods for him recently and she recalls that they did go out to a Mexican restaurant yesterday where he was fed corn for the first time and fava beans. He has a history of prolonged neonatal jaundice.

See pages 30–31 for answers

ANSWERS

Bowel conditions 1

1. G. Large bowel obstruction
X-ray typically shows bowel dilation proximal to the site of obstruction and collapse distal to it.

2. C. Crohn's disease
This patient has abdominal pain associated with diarrhoea for a prolonged period of time, he has barium enema evidence of Crohn's and a biopsy reveals a non-caseating granuloma which is seen in Crohn's disease but not ulcerative colitis.

3. K. Small bowel obstruction
This patient has classic features of small bowel obstruction including high pitched bowel sounds, distended small bowel loops and multiple air fluid levels.

4. E. Irritable bowel syndrome
This patient has symptoms for at least one day a week for at least three months, this is associated with relief with defecation, changes in stool frequency and change in form. She meets all the Rome IV diagnostic criteria for IBS.

5. H. Meckel's diverticulum
This is an outpouching in the small intestine, most people with this condition are asymptomatic but usually present with painless rectal bleeding if symptomatic.

Bowel conditions 2

1. B. Carcinoid syndrome
This condition occurs when a rare cancerous tumor secretes excessive amounts of serotonin into your blood stream.

2. I. Ogilvie syndrome
This condition is as a result of an acute dilatation of the colon, the caecum is commonly involved, without existing mechanical obstruction. It is a common presentation in the post-partum period particularly after caesarean section. If left untreated it can result in bowel perforation.

3. N. Toxic megacolon
This condition is typically associated with ulcerative colitis. Patients usually present with abdominal distension, fever and abdominal pain. Abdominal X-ray reveals an enlarged and distended transverse colon.

4. F. Ischaemic colitis
This condition involves inflammatory changes in the colon as a result of vascular insufficiency. This condition is mostly found in the elderly and is the most common type of bowel ischemia. Abdominal X-ray may show the characteristic "thumbprint" sign.

5. A. Bowel perforation
This patient has presented with acute abdominal pain with free air under the diaphragm which suggests perforation.

Bowel conditions 3

1. L. Small intestinal bacterial overgrowth
The gold standard for SIBO diagnosis is quantitative culture of a jejunal aspirate but glucose hydrogen breath testing can be used as a non-invasive alternative. Glucose hydrogen breath test can be used to diagnose SIBO if there is a rise in breath hydrogen.

2. M. Short gut syndrome
This condition is caused by either surgical resection or disease of the small bowel. Patients usually suffer from severe diarrhoea and weight loss as a result of malabsorption.

3. D. Diverticulitis
In this condition there is inflammation in small pouches of bowel known as diverticula which can develop in the large bowel. Patients commonly present with left lower quadrant pain and a fever.

4. O. Ulcerative colitis
In this condition there are inflammatory changes in the large bowel and rectum. Colonoscopy reveals continuous mucosal inflammation starting at the anal verge and extending up to a portion of or the entirety of the large bowel.

5. J. Pseudomembranous colitis
The correct answer is pseudomembranous colitis. This condition is caused by overgrowth of *Clostridium difficile* after commencement of antibiotic treatment.

Esophageal disorders 1

1. K. Viral esophagitis
This patient is immunocompromised and has presented with flu like symptoms associated with chest pain and odynophagia. Endoscopy reveals ulceration which is likely consistent with herpes simplex virus.

2. J. Mallory–Weiss tear
Mallory–Weiss tears occur in the lower section of the esophagus, these tears are most commonly caused by violent episodes of vomiting. Alcohol consumption is a contributing factor.

3. G. Esophageal cancer
This patient presents with dysphagia, odynophagia, weight loss, loss of appetite and likely has recurrent laryngeal nerve involvement. Patients typically have difficulty with swallowing solids initially and then fluids as obstruction worsens.

4. B. Barrett's esophagus
Barrett's esophagus results from acid reflux which damages the esophageal lining, this causes the lining to become red and thick. Barrett's esophagus is a common feature in patients with scleroderma.

5. H. Esophageal varices
This patient has presented with haematemesis and evidence of chronic liver disease. Esophageal varices are enlarged veins in the esophagus which commonly occur as a result of portal hypertension in severe liver disease.

Esophageal disorders 2

1. A. Achalasia
Achalasia is a condition which results in impaired peristalsis in the esophagus and failure of the ring-shaped musculature at the bottom of the esophagus to relax, resulting in a rat's tail or bird's beak appearance seen with barium swallow.
2. I. Gastroesophageal reflux disease
This patient has typical reflux symptoms which occur at least twice a week.
3. E. Eosinophilic esophagitis
This is an inflammatory condition of the esophagus. This patient has evidence of esophageal dysfunction and has classic features seen on endoscopy. Biopsy with greater or equal to 15 eosinophils per high-powered field is diagnostic.
4. D. Diffuse esophageal spasm
In this condition there is disorganised contraction of the esophagus which can result in chest pain, dysphagia and regurgitation of food. Barium swallow reveals a characteristic corkscrew appearance within the esophagus.
5. F. Esophageal candidiasis
It is likely that this patient's symptoms are as a result of inhaled corticosteroids, this is an important complication that patients must be aware of.

Gastric disorders 1

1. D. Gastric cancer
This patient is suffering from gastrointestinal symptoms, has a loss of weight, loss of appetite and epigastric discomfort. The barium swallow is suggestive of linitis plastica.
2. A. Coeliac disease
This is an autoimmune condition in which the body's immune system reacts to gluten. The gold standard for diagnosis is endoscopy and biopsy of the duodenum. Diagnosis is confirmed when biopsy demonstrates characteristic intra-epithelial lymphocytosis with blunting of villi.
3. B. Dumping syndrome
In this condition food passes from the stomach into the small bowel rapidly, especially high sugar content food. This results in hypoglycaemia which manifests with symptoms such as sweats, palpitations, light headedness, tremors anxiety and confusion to name a few. This condition can occur after weight loss related gastric surgery.
4. H. Hiatus hernia
A Hiatal hernia occurs when the upper part of the stomach bulges through the diaphragm into the chest cavity. A chest X-ray typically reveals a well-defined retrocardiac opacity with an air-fluid level.

Gastric disorders 2

1. C. Duodenal ulcers

These ulcers develop in the first part of the small intestine known as the duodenum. Pain associated with this is usually persistent and can be relieved by eating.

2. E. Gastric ulcer

These ulcers occur as a result of a break in the lining of the stomach. Helicobacter pylori is and NSAID use are common causes.

3. I. Perforated peptic ulcer

The initial symptom of this is usually sudden onset severe epigastric pain which persists and is made worse with movement and Valsalva. Erect abdominal or chest X-ray reveals free air under the diaphragm.

4. F. Gastroenteritis

Gastroenteritis is a condition which can present with fevers, sweats, myalgia, diarrhoea, vomiting, nausea and abdominal pains. It is commonly caused by viral and bacterial agents but can result from parasites and medication also.

Gastrointestinal conditions (Paediatric) 1

1. I. Pyloric stenosis

This condition causes blockage of food within the stomach and prevention of its entry into the duodenum. On examination an olive shaped lump may be palpable in the epigastrium which represents an enlarged pylorus. Pyloric stenosis can result in forceful vomiting, dehydration and loss of weight.

2. F. Meconium ileus

In this condition meconium (a child's first stool) blocks the last part of the small intestine (ileum). This condition is usually one of the earliest manifestations of cystic fibrosis.

3. C. Gastroenteritis

Gastroenteritis is a condition which can present with fevers, sweats, myalgia, diarrhoea, vomiting, nausea and abdominal pains. It is commonly caused by viral and bacterial agents but can result from parasites and medication also.

4. E. Intussusception

This child presents with classic features including red currant jelly stools, abdominal mass and intermittent abdominal discomfort. The mass is formed as a result of invagination of the proximal small bowel segment into the distal segment of the small intestine.

5. A. Appendicitis

This patient has presented with classic features of acute appendicitis with migratory pain and tenderness in the right lower quadrant, this requires urgent surgical review.

6. K. Wilm's tumor

Also known as a nephroblastoma, this is the most common type of kidney cancer in children.

Gastrointestinal conditions (Paediatric) 2

1. D. Hirschsprung's disease

This child has not passaged meconium since birth, they also have symptoms consistent with bowel obstruction. The child also has clinical features of Down syndrome, a condition commonly associated with Hirschsprung's disease.

2. J. Sigmoid volvulus

This condition is rare in the pediatric population and may cause bowel obstruction. A coffee bean appearance of the sigmoid bowel on abdominal X-ray is diagnostic.

3. G. Mesenteric adenitis

Mesenteric adenitis is a condition in which the lymph nodes of the abdomen enlarge, this condition can mimic acute appendicitis but typically the individual has a viral illness prior to commencement of symptoms.

4. H. Necrotising enterocolitis

This condition affects premature infants. Pneumatosis intestinalis (intramural bowel gas) is diagnostic for necrotising enterocolitis.

5. B. Duodenal atresia

Patients with this condition typically present on day one after birth with vomiting, bilious or non-bilious. X-ray shows the characteristic double bubble sign (air trapped in the stomach and duodenum, separated by the pyloric sphincter). During pregnancy a fetus with duodenal atresia causes increased amniotic fluid (polyhydramnios) as it interferes with gastrointestinal absorption of amniotic fluid swallowed by the fetus distal to the level of intestinal obstruction. Down syndrome is commonly associated with duodenal atresia.

Gastrointestinal imaging 1

1. G. Impending abdominal aortic aneurysm rupture

This sign is caused by blood which haemorrhages into the wall of the aneurysm or within the mural thrombus.

2. K. Pyloric stenosis

This describes the distended stomach with wave like contours which appear similar to a caterpillar.

3. F. Duodenal atresia

The left sided bubble represents the distended stomach, filled by fluid and air. The right sided bubble represents the distended duodenum.

4. B. Colorectal carcinoma.

The sign results from constriction of the lumen of the colon by an annular carcinoma.

5. N. Small bowel obstruction

This sign is created by gas trapped between the valvulae conniventes along the superior wall of dilated loops of small bowel.

Gastrointestinal imaging 2

1. A. Achalasia

This refers to the tapering of the inferior esophagus in this condition.

2. **L. Sigmoid volvulus**

This represents a U shaped, distended sigmoid colon.

3. **D. Diaphragmatic rupture**

This results from the constriction of the part of the liver which herniates through the diaphragm.

4. **I. Intussusception**

The sign is caused by a hypoechoic ring with central echogenicity.

5. **O. Ulcerative colitis**

This sign results from loss of the normal haustral pattern of the transverse, descending and sigmoid colon.

Gastrointestinal imaging 3

1. **M. Small bowel haematoma**

This is formed by small bowel folds which are uniformly thickened.

2. **J. Pneumoperitoneum**

The appearance results from a triangle of gas which forms between the abdominal wall and two bowel loops or three loops of bowel.

3. **E. Diffuse esophageal spasm**

This is a classic finding of diffuse esophageal spasm and reflects abnormal contractions resulting in compartmentalisation and curling of the esophagus.

4. **C. Crohn's disease**

It results from involvement of the stomach in Crohn's disease. The stomach becomes conical and more rigid giving the appearance of a ram's horn.

Hepatobiliary Disease 1

1. **C. Cholecystitis**

This is inflammation of the gall bladder. Murphy's sign is typically positive as the inflamed gall bladder presses against the examiner's hand on examination.

2. **D. Choledocholithiasis**

This occurs when the common bile duct contains a gall stone, this can cause jaundice and liver damage.

3. **K. Hepatitis B – chronic**

This patient has evidence of chronic infection serologically.

4. **M. Pancreatic cancer**

This patient has a palpable mass over the pancreas, they have a loss of weight/appetite and have clinical evidence of biliary obstruction.

5. **J. Hepatitis B–acute**

This patient has evidence of acute infection clinically and serologically.

Hepatobiliary Disease 2

1. **I. Hepatitis A**

This condition is very common in returned travellers and symptoms typically occur at two to four weeks after catching hepatitis A. Symptoms can include fever, nausea, abdominal discomfort, jaundice and dark coloured urine. Patients usually fully recover after an episode

2. A. Alcoholic hepatitis

This condition occurs as a result of excessive alcohol consumption. This patient shows evidence of liver failure on clinical examination and serology.

3. L. Hepatitis B–resolved

This patient has serological evidence of past infection which is no longer active.

4. N. Pancreatitis

This patient has presented with severe epigastric pain, vomiting and a lipase level at least three times the upper limit of normal.

Hepatobiliary Disease 3

1. O. Primary biliary cirrhosis

This patient presents with classic features of this condition and positive anti-mitochondrial antibodies.

2. P. Primary sclerosing cholangitis

This is a condition that involves inflammation and scarring of the bile ducts. Patients usually present with evidence of liver disease. Diagnosis is based on an elevated ALP, ERCP with characteristic beading pattern (caused by alternating strictures and dilations) and liver biopsy.

3. G. Gilbert's syndrome

This condition causes unconjugated hyperbilirubinemia in otherwise healthy individuals with normal liver function test results. The episodes of jaundice associated with Gilbert's syndrome are usually preceded by viral illness or stressful events.

4. H. Haemochromatosis

Patients usually present with fatigue and arthralgia initially but can progress to liver disease with more severe iron overload. A serum ferritin in a postmenopausal woman >300 µg/L and a transferrin saturation > 55% should raise suspicion of haemochromatosis.

5. B. Ascending cholangitis

This patient demonstrates Charcot's triad which is a combination of fever, jaundice and right upper quadrant pain. Murphy's sign is usually negative in ascending cholangitis.

Lumps and Hernias 1

1. B. Divarication of recti

In this condition there is thinning and widening of the linea alba. Valsalva can cause the midline to bulge.

2. J. Umbilical hernia

These mostly commonly occur in infants below the age of six months. The swelling in the umbilical region typically worsens with crying, coughing or straining.

3. F. Paraumbilical hernia

These types of hernias protrude above or below the umbilicus and are commonly found in adults.

4. E. Indirect inguinal hernia

With this type of hernia, when the examiner places pressure over the inguinal canal and asks the patient to perform a Valsalva manoeuvre the examiner will feel the bulge against their hand.

Lumps and Hernias 2

1. C. Epigastric hernia

They are located in the epigastric region, between the umbilicus and the xiphisternum. These hernias are usually small and of little concern, they can be present from birth and the majority of people with them are unaware that they have one.

2. H. Saphena varix

This results from dilatation of the saphenous vein and can easily be mistaken for an inguinal hernia, but disappears on lying flat.

3. A. Direct inguinal hernia

With this type of hernia if the examiner places pressure over the deep inguinal ring after reduction and asks the patient to perform a Valsalva manoeuvre the examiner will feel it protrude.

4. D. Femoral hernia

The neck of the femoral hernia is located below and lateral to the pubic tubercle as opposed to the inguinal hernia which is located above and medial to the pubic tubercle.

Perianal Conditions 1

1. H. Proctalgia fugax

This condition is a diagnosis of exclusion, often attributed to cramping of the anal sphincter complex.

2. B. Condyloma

This patient has presented with anal warts which typically present initially as pinhead sized growths and can slowly enlarge. Anal warts are caused by HPV and are the most common form of STI.

3. C. Internal haemorrhoid

These are found within the rectum above the dentate line, are painless as they are viscerally innervated but do tend to bleed.

4. G. Pilonidal sinus

This is a small hole or tunnel that typically forms in the natal cleft. They are usually of no concern unless they become infected.

5. A. Anal fissure

This is a small tear in the skin that surrounds the anus. In this case the most likely cause is constipation.

6. I. Rectal prolapse

Patients typically describe a bulge protruding from the anus. It is caused by weakened muscles that support the rectum and is commonly associated with constipation and traumatic events such as childbirth.

Perianal Conditions 2

1. D. Molluscum contagiosum

This is an infection caused by a poxvirus. The typical finding is flesh coloured bumps which are round and dimpled in their centres. They are common in children and are regarded as an STI in adults.

2. F. Perianal haematoma

This is a lump that is formed by a ruptured or bleeding vein that causes a collection in the tissue around the anus. It typically appears as a blue lump under the skin. It is sometimes referred to as an external haemorrhoid.

3. J. Rectal varices

This patient likely has portal hypertension as a result of liver disease caused by alcoholism. Rectal varices are a complication of portal hypertension.

4. K. Solitary rectal ulcer syndrome

This is a rare condition commonly caused by chronic constipation which causes internal rectal intussusception. The rectal lining gets damaged by friction, this results in ulceration.

5. E. Perianal abscess

This is a superficial infection which causes a lump to form around the anus, this lump is formed by the build-up of pus. The lump is very tender and can cause difficulty sitting down.

Paediatric jaundice 1

1. D. Cephalohematoma*

Blood in a cephalohematoma is broken down and leads to an elevation of bilirubin as such children born with these are at an increased risk of jaundice.

2. I. Galactosaemia

This is a life-threatening condition in which a newborn is unable to metabolise galactose which is found in breast milk and dairy products.

3. L. Physiological jaundice

This commonly occurs two to four days after delivery in a term infant.

4. A. ABO incompatibility

In ABO haemolytic disease of the newborn IgG antibodies from the mother which are specific for ABO blood group pass to the fetal circulation via the placenta and cause hemolysis of the fetal red blood cells and anaemia.

Paediatric jaundice 2

1. K. Hypothyroidism

This patient presents with symptoms of congenital hypothyroidism which include excessive sleepiness, jaundice, constipation, large tongue and dry skin.

2. B. Biliary atresia

In this condition there is a blockage of the ducts that lead out of the liver, these ducts carry bile from the liver to the gallbladder. This condition occurs because there is poor development of these bile ducts. The triangular cord sign is positive if there is increased echogenicity along the anterior wall of the portal vein. The triangular cord sign represents a fibrous ductal remnant of the extrahepatic bile duct. This patient also has a small gall bladder, less than 19 mm in length.

3. C. Breast milk jaundice

This usually presents a few days into the first week after delivery. The child has elevated unconjugated hyperbilirubinemia but is otherwise well and healthy. The jaundice usually resolves spontaneously.

4. J. G6PD Deficiency

This patient has presented with favism, a clinical syndrome that results from consumption of fava beans. This syndrome results in acute haemolytic anaemia.

Dermatology

2

CHILDHOOD INFECTIONS 1

A. Chicken pox
B. Erythema infectiosum
C. Hand, foot and mouth disease
D. Kawasaki syndrome
E. Measles
F. Molluscum contagiosum
G. Mumps
H. Rheumatic fever
I. Roseola infantum
J. Rubella
K. Scarlet fever
L. Staphylococcal scalded skin syndrome

For each of the following, what is the MOST likely diagnosis?

1. A 6-year-old child presents with a sore throat, headache, fever and rash. On examination she has a temperature of 38.1°C, there is white exudate over bilateral tonsils. She has a blanching erythematous rash which covers her axillae, chest and neck and has a sandpaper like texture to it.
2. A 6-year-old girl presents with a red rash on her cheeks. She has felt unwell for the past two days and has had a mild fever and headache. On examination she has a temperature of 36.2°C and bright red cheeks bilaterally.
3. A 2-year-old child attends with a two-day history of sores in his mouth which have been causing him difficulty with eating. On examination there are ulcers in the buccal and labial mucosa. You also note flat pink patches on the palms of the hands and red papules in the natal cleft.
4. A 7-year-old girl presents to your clinic with a blistering rash. Her mother explains that they started out as itchy red dots but have now become blisters. On examination there are scattered vesicles on the back, abdomen and face.
5. A 4-year-old boy presents after his mother noticed papular lesions on his abdomen. He has not had any recent illness and his mother reports that he is otherwise well today. On examination there are clusters of shiny small

DOI: 10.1201/9781003459941-2

round papules, with umbilicated centres. His 3-year-old sister has similar lesions.

6. A 6-year-old girl presents with a five-day history of fever. She also complains of joint pain in her ankles, knees, elbows and wrists. She had an episode of tonsillitis two week ago. On examination she has a temperature of 39.2°C, you note erythema marginatum on the trunks and upper limbs, there are also subcutaneous nodules in the elbows. Laboratory investigations reveal an elevated CRP of 102 and an ECG demonstrates PR prolongation.

See page 48 for answers.

CHILDHOOD INFECTIONS 2

A. Chicken pox
B. Erythema infectiosum
C. Hand, foot and mouth disease
D. Kawasaki syndrome
E. Measles
F. Molluscum contagiosum
G. Mumps
H. Rheumatic fever
I. Roseola infantum
J. Rubella
K. Scarlet fever
L. Staphylococcal scalded skin syndrome

For each of the following, what is the MOST likely diagnosis?

1. A 4-year-old boy presents with a one-day history of central chest pain in the context of a five-day history of fever. On examination he has a temperature of 39.1°C, a polymorphous rash, cervical lymphadenopathy, bilateral conjunctivitis and a strawberry tongue.

2. An 8-year-old girl presents with a 24-hour history of non-itchy rash. Her mother explains that the rash started behind her ears and on her face and spread to the rest of the body. She has also been suffering from conjunctivitis for the past two days and a fever which started today. On examination she has a temperature of 38.4°C, there are flat red spots covering the back, trunk and limbs but sparing the palms and soles. On oral examination you note Koplik spots opposite the molars.

3. A 3-year-old girl attends with her mother who is very worried about a widespread, macular, erythematous rash she noticed this morning. She has had a fever for the past four days. On examination she is smiling and has a temperature of 36.5°C, the rash is widespread and blanching.

4. A 1-week-old child presents to your emergency department with her concerned parents. She has been irritable, has had a fever for the past 24 hours and a rash has appeared on her body last night. On examination she has a temperature of 38.3°C, there widespread redness with peeling of the top layer of the skin, bullae in the axillae and bilateral groin regions. Nikolsky sign is positive.

5. An 11-year-old boy presents with fever and painful swelling in bilateral cheeks. He is an unaccompanied minor and has recently arrived as a refugee from Syria. Through an interpreter he explains that he has had a headache for a couple of days before the swelling commenced and he has been struggling to eat and talk. He has not had any childhood vaccinations.

See page 48 for answers.

SKIN REACTIONS

A. **Acute generalised exanthematous pustulosis**
B. **Congenital erythropoietic protoporphyria**
C. **DRESS syndrome**
D. **Erythropoietic protoporphyria**
E. **Fixed drug eruption**
F. **Jarisch–Herxheimer reaction**
G. **Porphyria cutanea tarda**
H. **Stevens–Johnson syndrome**
I. **Variegate porphyria**

For each of the following, what is the MOST likely diagnosis?

1. A 44-year-old presents with a five-day history of generalised rash and facial swelling. On examination she has a temperature of 38.1°C, morbilliform rash affecting the entire body, hepatomegaly and generalised lymphadenopathy. Nikolsky sign is negative. Laboratory investigations reveal an elevated bilirubin, transaminase at greater than four times the upper limit of normal, leukocytosis and a differential leukocyte count revealing eosinophilia. She commenced lamotrigine six weeks ago for management of newly diagnosed epilepsy.

2. A 48-year-old attends with a chronic history of blistering rash on the back of his hands and forearms. His symptoms commence after sun exposure and are particularly bad on hot days. He has also noticed that his urine has been dark in color. He reports that he drinks six standard drinks on weekend days and has done so for the past 10 years. On examination there is a blistering rash over the forearms and dorsal surfaces of the hands. A urine sample is collected which is tea colored. Examination of the urine with Wood's lamp reveals a coral pink fluorescence. Laboratory investigations reveal high levels of porphyrin in his stools, urine and circulating red cells.

3. A 27-year-old presents with tonsillitis, you commence her on a course of phenoxymethylpenicillin. The next day she returns to your clinic with a pruritic rash which started on the face and groin then rapidly spread to the rest of the body. On examination she has a temperature of 38.2°C, you note diffusely erythematous skin covered in pinhead sized, non-follicular pustules. She also has swelling in her face. You cease the phenoxymethylpenicillin and refer her to the local emergency department. Eight days later the skin peels and the rash resolves.

4. A 31-year-old presents with a sore on his penis and inguinal lymph node enlargement. You arrange for laboratory investigations which confirm that he has syphilis and you subsequently commence IM benzathine benzylpenicillin. He returns to your clinic the next morning complaining of a rash, fever, joint pain and nausea. On examination he has a diffuse monomorphic papular rash across his trunk and extremities.

5. A 34-year-old presents with an itchy rash on her right lower abdomen. You saw her yesterday for a chest infection and commenced her on amoxicillin. On examination there is a single well defined, oval shaped violaceous blistering plaque. She reports that she had a similar presentation three years prior after a course of amoxicillin.

6. A 32-year-old HIV positive male presents with a fever and chesty cough for the past three days. On examination he has a temperature of 38.6°C and bronchial breath sounds in bilateral lower zones. You arrange for a sputum MCS which returns positive for *P. jirovecii* and he is subsequently started on a course of trimethoprim + sulfamethoxazole. He returns to your clinic five days later with painful erythematous lesions and blisters on his upper limbs and trunk. He also has blisters in his mouth and sore eyes. On examination there are areas where the blisters have merged to form sheets of skin detachment with underlying red dermis.

See pages 48–49 for answers.

HAIR

A. **Alopecia areata**
B. **Anagen effluvium**
C. **Androgenetic alopecia**
D. **Hirsutism**
E. **Hypertrichosis**
F. **Lichen planopilaris**
G. **Loose anagen syndrome**
H. **Telogen effluvium**
I. **Tinea capitis**
J. **Trichotillomania**

For each of the following, what is the MOST likely diagnosis?

1. A 36-year-old is concerned about excessive hair growth. He reports that he has had hair growing in odd locations including: over the dorsum of his hands, over his ears, across his back and over his anterior neck. This has caused him much embarrassment and he is constantly having to remove the hair.

2. A 24-year-old is concerned about hair loss. She explains that she was having her hair done for her upcoming graduation and her hairdresser discovered a bald patch on her head. She has no significant past medical history and is not using any regular medications. On examination there is a well-defined circular bald patch on the right side of her head with normal skin. Dermoscopic examination reveals exclamation mark hairs at the edge.

3. A 41-year-old presents with generalised hair loss. She has no significant medical history and takes no regular medications. Two months ago, she was hospitalised for severe pneumonia and reports that she is otherwise well. On examination there is a positive hair pull test on the vertex and scalp margins. The modified wash test is also positive for club shedding hair.

4. An 8-year-old girl presents with hair loss on her head which has been present for the past three months. She has seen several GPs and has tried a variety of topical and oral agents without success. On examination there is patchy hair loss, broken hair ends of varying lengths and hair powder. Her mother is very distressed as she has been following this up on her own as she recently separated from her partner who has moved interstate.

5. A 23-year-old woman presents concerned about excessive hair growth. Since she was a teenager has had thick hair growth in her armpits, groin and across her face. Her symptoms have caused her much social embarrassment and distress.

6. A 6-year-old boy presents with an itchy scalp for the past four weeks associated with some hair loss. On examination there are several small sharply defined circular lesions with hair loss on the scalp. Trichoscopy demonstrates multiple comma shaped hairs. Wood's lamp exam demonstrates green fluorescence on the lesions.

See page 49 for answers.

NAILS 1

A. **Acrolentiginous melanoma**
B. **Acute paronychia**
C. **Alopecia areata**
D. **Candida onychia**
E. **Chronic paronychia**
F. **Darier disease**
G. **Felon**

H. Green nail syndrome
I. Lichen planus
J. Longitudinal melanonychia
K. Myxoid cyst
L. Onychauxis
M. Onychogryphosis
N. Onycholysis
O. Panchyonychia congenita
P. Psoriasis
Q. Subungual hematoma

For each of the following, what is the MOST likely diagnosis?

1. A 31-year-old presents with a black discoloration in her left great toe. It has been there for the past four weeks and she is not happy with the appearance. On examination there is a well-defined black discoloration affecting the lateral lower half of her left great toe. Dermoscopic examination reveals a roundish shape with peripheral fading and linear white marks on the nail plate. She explains that she dropped a 5 kg weight on her toe shortly before the discoloration appeared.

2. An 18-month-old is struggling to walk. On examination there is thickening of the skin in the soles of her feet and the palms of her hand. You also observe thickening and brown discoloration of the nails.

3. A 32-year-old presents with a six-month history of brittle nails. She has also been suffering from dry skin on her left elbow but she is managing well with over-the-counter treatments. On examination you note pitting of the nails, oil spots on the nail beds and punctate leukonychia. There are also two silver-white scaly patches on her left elbow with mild erythema.

4. A 56-year-old presents with a lump in his right index finger which has been present for the past six months. On examination there is a semi-translucent lesion with a shiny surface on the dorsum of the right index finger involving the proximal nail fold. He tried to remove it at home and a jelly like fluid has come out of it and then it grew back.

5. A 24-year-old presents with painful swelling in his left index finger. He jammed the finger while at work and the symptoms developed by the end of the day. On examination there is erythema in the proximal nail fold with associated yellow pus under the cuticle.

See pages 49–50 for answers.

NAILS 2

A. Acrolentiginous melanoma
B. Acute paronychia
C. Alopecia areata
D. Candida onychia
E. Chronic paronychia
F. Darier disease
G. Felon
H. Green nail syndrome
 I. Lichen planus
 J. Longitudinal melanonychia
K. Myxoid cyst
L. Onychauxis
M. Onychogryphosis
N. Onycholysis
O. Panchyonychia congenita
P. Psoriasis
Q. Subungual hematoma

For each of the following, what is the MOST likely diagnosis?

1. A 24-year-old presents with a six-month history of "nail lifting". She first noticed it in her right index finger but it has now spread to other nails in bilateral hands. On examination the distal part of the affected nails appears greyish-white in color and is not attached to the distal nail bed.
2. A 28-year-old HIV positive male presents with discoloration in his nails. On examination there are white longitudinal streaks in the nail plates and nail thickening.
3. An 82-year-old man presents for his annual diabetes review. On examination of his toes, you note that the great toe on his left foot is severely distorted, thickened and has a ram's hornlike deformity.
4. A 67-year-old presents with worsening brown discoloration in the left great toe for the past three months. On examination there are dark brown parallel lines in the lateral aspect of the left great toe and a notable Hutchinson sign.
5. A 37-year-old complains of a three-month history of worsening painless right index finger swelling. She has seen several GPs who have tried various antibiotics without success. On examination the nail is disfigured, there is inflammation of the proximal and lateral nail folds, the proximal nail fold is retracted and the cuticle is absent.

See page 50 for answers.

NAIL SIGNS OF SYSTEMIC ILLNESS

A. **Apparent leukonychia**
B. **Beau's lines**
C. **Koilonychia**
D. **Periungual erythema**
E. **Periungual fibroma**
F. **Pterygium inversum unguium**
G. **Splinter haemorrhages**
H. **Yellow nail syndrome**

For each of the following, what is the MOST likely diagnosis?

1. A 42-year-old presents to your clinic for a referral to see his hepatologist. He has a history of liver cirrhosis secondary to chronic hepatitis B infection and has six monthly reviews with his specialist. On examination you note that the proximal two-thirds of his nail plates appear white and the distal third shows the red color of the nailbed.

2. A 28-year-old presents with fatigue. She is a vegan and has a history of menorrhagia. On examination you note that her fingernail plates are concave in shape.

3. A 38-year-old woman attends your outpatient clinic for review. She is currently undergoing chemotherapy for breast cancer. She reports that she has been well. She examines well but you note that there are transverse, band like ridges in all of her nails.

4. A 39-year-old presents with enlarging abnormal nail growths. She has a history of tuberous sclerosis and has had no recent medication changes. On examination there are several skin-colored lesions arising from the proximal nail folds which are associated with longitudinal grooves in the nail plates.

5. A 38-year-old explains that his nails have "stopped growing". He reports that he has also noticed swelling in his legs but is otherwise well. He has a history of recurrent pleural effusions and you have seen him several times for chest infections. On examination he has thickened nails which are greenish-yellow in color, you also note lymphoedema in his lower limbs.

See pages 50–51 for answers.

DERMATITIS 1

A. **Allergic contact dermatitis**
B. **Asteatotic dermatitis**
C. **Atopic dermatitis**

D. **Brachioradial pruritus**
E. **Dermatitis artefacta**
F. **Dyshidrotic eczematous dermatitis**
G. **Irritant contact dermatitis**
H. **Lichen simplex chronicus**
I. **Nummular eczema**
J. **Prurigo nodularis**
K. **Seborrheic dermatitis**
L. **Terra firma-forme dermatosis**

For each of the following, what is the MOST likely diagnosis?

1. A 53-year-old man presents with an intensely itchy lesion on the right side of his back just below the scapula. He reports that it has been irritating him for the past 10 years and would like to have a referral to see a dermatologist. He has no significant medical history. On examination there is an irregular red plaque with a significant amount of lichenification.

2. A 58-year-old man presents with a four-month history of itchy rash on his shins which is associated with areas of dry scaly skin. He reports that his symptoms slowly worsened with time. He also explains that his symptoms are particularly worse on cold days. On examination there are diamond shaped plates separated by red lines giving a "crazy-paving" appearance.

3. A 39-year-old man attends for review of a chronic, non-itchy rash affecting his face. He has no significant medical history. On examination there is a yellowish coloured greasy scale surrounded by salmon pink skin over his eyebrows, moustache and in his nasolabial folds.

4. A 54-year-old woman presents with an itchy rash on her arms and hands which started a few hours after gardening. She explains that she had a similar rash four weeks ago when she was gardening but to a lesser extent. On examination there is well demarcated erythema and peeling of the skin in bilateral hands and on her right forearm.

See page 51 for answers.

DERMATITIS 2

A. **Allergic contact dermatitis**
B. **Asteatotic dermatitis**
C. **Atopic dermatitis**
D. **Brachioradial pruritus**
E. **Dermatitis artefacta**
F. **Dyshidrotic eczematous dermatitis**
G. **Irritant contact dermatitis**

H. Lichen simplex chronicus
 I. Nummular eczema
 J. Prurigo nodularis
K. Seborrheic dermatitis
 L. Terra firma-forme dermatosis

For each of the following, what is the MOST likely diagnosis?

1. A 19-year-old presents with an itchy rash on his hands, he also reports a burning sensation at times. He explains that he has had flare-ups of these symptoms for the past 12 months. On examination there are crops of deep-seated blisters covering both hands, there is also fissure formation on the palms.
2. A 22-year-old presents with recurrent flares of itchy rash affecting his axillae, cubital and popliteal fossae. He is an asthmatic and uses Ventolin as required. On examination there are erythematous lesions in the areas of concern, there is also associated exudate.
3. A 26-year-old woman complains of an itchy rash affecting bilateral lower limbs for the past week which is progressively worsening. On examination there are several well-defined coin shaped plaques across the thighs bilaterally, each measuring between 2–3 cm in diameter.
4. A 23-year-old trainee hairdresser attends your clinic complaining of a two-day history of burning sensation and pain in his hands. He explains that he has never had symptoms like this before and they began shortly after washing the hair of a client with a shampoo he has never used. On examination there is erythema and blistering on both of his palms.

See page 51 for answers.

INFLAMMATORY DISORDERS 1

A. Chronic superficial scaly dermatitis
B. Doucas–Kapetanakis eczematid-like purpura
C. Erythema multiforme
D. Erythema nodosum
E. Granuloma annulare
 F. Granuloma faciale
G. Lichen aureus
H. Lichen planus
 I. Morphea
 J. Pityriasis lichenoides et varioliformis acuta
K. Pityriasis rosea
 L. Purpura annularis telangiectodes
M. Pyoderma gangrenosum

N. Schamberg disease
O. Sweet's syndrome

For each of the following, what is the MOST likely diagnosis?

1. A 5-year-old presents with a lesion on her hand which has been present for the past four weeks and has not gone away. She has not been scratching at it and it does not seem to bother her. On examination there is a flesh-coloured raised ring-like lesion over the dorsum of the right PIP of the index finger. The surface of the lesion is smooth and the centre is slightly depressed.

2. A 67-year-old woman presents with a painful ulcerating lesion over her left shin. She explains that she pricked her shin on a rose bush while gardening, the next day noticed a small red bump which rapidly developed into an ulcer. On examination there is an ulcer on her shin with a violaceous border.

3. A 60-year-old man presents with tender bumps on his left hand which are progressively increasing. On examination there are multiple red-purple nodules and vesicles on the dorsum of his left hand and thumb. On palpation the lesions are solid. A biopsy is performed which reveals dense neutrophilic infiltration in the papillary dermis without evidence of vasculitis.

4. A 26-year-old woman attends with a pruritic rash affecting her right wrist. On examination there are several purple, flat topped, shiny, polygonal plaques over her right wrist. The plaques are crossed by fine white lines.

See pages 51–52 for answers.

INFLAMMATORY DISORDERS 2

A. Chronic superficial scaly dermatitis
B. Doucas–Kapetanakis eczematid-like purpura
C. Erythema multiforme
D. Erythema nodosum
E. Granuloma annulare
F. Granuloma faciale
G. Lichen aureus
H. Lichen planus
I. Morphea
J. Pityriasis lichenoides et varioliformis acuta
K. Pityriasis rosea
L. Purpura annularis telangiectodes
M. Pyoderma gangrenosum
N. Schamberg disease
O. Sweet's syndrome

For each of the following, what is the MOST likely diagnosis?

1. A 19-year-old woman attends your clinic complaining of a widespread non-pruritic rash which has been present for the past two days. On examination she has multiple scaly oval shaped lesions across her chest and back which resemble a Christmas tree in distribution. She attended your clinic two weeks ago because she noticed a single large circular lesion on her abdomen.

2. A 14-year-old girl attends your GP clinic concerned about a discoloration over the right side of her forehead which has been present for the past six months. She denies any associated pain or itch. On examination there is a linear, hyperpigmented patch over the right forehead extending from the lateral eyebrow to her hairline.

3. A 25-year-old woman presents to your clinic with painful red nodules over her anterior shins. You saw her two weeks ago for tonsillitis which you treated with penicillin. On examination there are several tender erythematous nodules measuring between 3–5 cm in diameter over the anterior surfaces of bilateral shins.

4. A 32-year-old man presents with pruritic lesions on his hands and feet which have now spread onto his torso. He explains that three days ago he had ulceration in his mouth and around his lip which is still present. On examination you note numerous small target lesions on his hands, feet and torso.

See page 52 for answers.

SKIN LESIONS 1

A. **Actinic keratoses**
B. **Basal cell carcinoma**
C. **Chondrodermatitis nodularis helicis**
D. **Dermatofibroma**
E. **Dermatofibrosarcoma protuberans**
F. **Gorlin syndrome**
G. **Invasive squamous cell carcinoma**
H. **Keratoacanthoma**
I. **Merkel cell carcinoma**
J. **Myxoid cyst**
K. **Pilar cyst**
L. **Polymorphous light eruption**
M. **Pyogenic granuloma**
N. **Solar lentigo**
O. **Squamous cell carcinoma in situ**

For each of the following, what is the MOST likely diagnosis?

1. A 36-year-old woman presents with a lump on the crown of her head. The lesion has been present for the past five years but is now pruritic and has been worsening over the past 4 weeks. On examination there is a cystic structure measuring 2 cm x 2 cm without a central punctum.

2. A 66-year-old is concerned about a rapidly growing lesion on his nose. On examination there is a 2.5 cm well defined, round, erythematous lesion with a central hyperkeratotic plug.

3. A 71-year-old farmer is concerned about a scaly rash on his face, forehead and hands. He explains that he initially had small scattered lesions which have gradually increased in size and number. On examination there is excessively dry appearing skin with multiple red-coloured scaly lesions on the face, forehead and hands. The lesions are tender to touch. A "strawberry" pattern appearance is evident on dermoscopy.

4. A 54-year-old farmer presents with a five-month history of a lesion on his right cheek which he is concerned about. On examination there is a well-defined pearly, nodular lesion with telangiectasia on its surface.

5. A 34-year-old is concerned about a painless lump on her left shin that has been present for the past 12 months. She explains that she is embarrassed by it and cannot wear skirts as a result, she has also caught it a few times while shaving her legs. On examination there is a solitary firm red-brown nodule on the left shin, pinch sign is positive.

6. A 61-year-old presents with a nine-month history of a slowly enlarging lesion on her right forearm. On examination there is an erythematous plaque with an irregular border measuring 3 cm in diameter. There is scaling on the surface of the lesion. Dermoscopy reveals irregular clusters of glomerular vessels.

See pages 52–53 for answers.

SKIN LESIONS 2

A. **Actinic keratoses**
B. **Basal cell carcinoma**
C. **Chondrodermatitis nodularis helicis**
D. **Dermatofibroma**
E. **Dermatofibrosarcoma protuberans**
F. **Gorlin syndrome**
G. **Invasive squamous cell carcinoma**
H. **Keratoacanthoma**
I. **Merkel cell carcinoma**
J. **Myxoid cyst**
K. **Pilar cyst**

L. Polymorphous light eruption
M. Pyogenic granuloma
N. Solar lentigo
O. Squamous cell carcinoma in situ

For each of the following, what is the MOST likely diagnosis?

1. A 26-year-old woman presents to your clinic concerned about a painless red lump on her right cheek. She gave birth one month ago and first noticed the lump in her final trimester of pregnancy. On examination there is a shiny red fleshy nodule over her right cheek which measures 1 cm in diameter.
2. A 37-year-old man presents with a lesion on the left side of his forehead. He explains that it bleeds easily even after gentle scraping. On examination there is a soft, dome shaped, red coloured nodule without hyperkeratosis.
3. A 26-year-old woman is concerned about a rash she has been suffering from. She explains that she has a rash across her face, chest and arms which develops every spring. On examination she has crops of pink papules across her cheeks, the V of her neck and her upper limbs.
4. A 46-year-old Caucasian woman presents to your clinic as she is concerned about a brown patch which has developed over the past 12 months on the dorsum of her right hand. On examination there is a well-defined, round, symmetrical, macular tan-brown lesion on the dorsum of her right hand.
5. A 31-year-old man presents to your clinic complaining of a four-month history of right ear swelling and discomfort which awakens him at night. On examination there is a firm, solitary, oval shaped lesion over the apex of the helix of the right pinna. There is associated central crust and surrounding erythema.

See page 53 for answers.

PIGMENTATION DISORDERS 1

A. Acanthosis nigricans
B. Albinism
C. Erythrasma
D. Melasma
E. Mongolian blue spot
F. Naevus anaemicus
G. Neurofibromatosis – type 1
H. Peutz–Jeghers syndrome
 I. Pityriasis alba
J. Pityriasis versicolor
K. Poikiloderma of Civatte
L. Seborrheic keratosis

M. **Superficial spreading melanoma**
N. **Tinea nigra**
O. **Trichomycosis axillaris**
P. **Tuberous sclerosis**
Q. **Vitiligo**

For each of the following, what is the MOST likely diagnosis?

1. A 32-year-old type 2 diabetic male presents to your clinic concerned about a rash in his right armpit which has been present for the past six months. On examination there is a well-defined brown patch in the right armpit with fine scaling. Wood's lamp examination demonstrates coral-pink fluorescence.

2. A 43-year-old woman presents with a 12-month history of red discoloration over her upper chest and neck. She reports that at times there is itching and burning sensations in the affected areas. She has no significant medical history and does not take any medication. On examination there are symmetrical, red coloured, atrophic patches over her upper chest and the sides of her neck with sparing of the submental area.

3. A 22-year-old man recently returned from a two-week holiday in Southern Spain and has noticed discoloration on his trunk and neck. On examination there are patches across the trunk and neck which are paler than surrounding tanned skin. The patches have a bran like scale.

4. A 3-year-old child presents with his parents who are concerned about hypopigmented lesions they have noticed on his body. He has a history of developmental delay and recurrent seizures for which he is seeing a paediatrician. On examination there are two hypomelanotic macular lesions on his chest and two on his back which are ash leaf–shaped.

5. A 36-year-old woman presents to your GP clinic with a worsening non-pruritic, non-painful, brown patch on her right hand. On examination there is an asymmetrical brown patch on her right palm which is slightly scaly. A biopsy is performed which demonstrates multiple short, segmented hyphae and spores in the stratum corneum which are brown coloured with H&E staining.

See page 53 for answers.

PIGMENTATION DISORDERS 2

A. **Acanthosis nigricans**
B. **Albinism**
C. **Erythrasma**
D. **Melasma**
E. **Mongolian blue spot**
F. **Naevus anaemicus**

G. **Neurofibromatosis – type 1**
H. **Peutz–Jeghers syndrome**
 I. **Pityriasis alba**
 J. **Pityriasis versicolor**
K. **Poikiloderma of Civatte**
L. **Seborrheic keratosis**
M. **Superficial spreading melanoma**
N. **Tinea nigra**
O. **Trichomycosis axillaris**
 P. **Tuberous sclerosis**
Q. **Vitiligo**

For each of the following, what is the MOST likely diagnosis?

1. A 3-year-old attends with his mother as she is concerned about a non-pruritic discoloration she has noticed on his face. On examination there are multiple circular hypopigmented patches across his face measuring between 0.5 and 1 cm in diameter.
2. A 36-year-old woman presents with dark brown discolouration across her face which has been present for the past four months. She is currently 36 weeks' gestation and has no significant medical history. On examination there are symmetrical, bilateral dark brown macules with irregular borders on the malar cheeks and forehead.
3. A 39-year-old woman presents to your clinic concerned about a lesion she has had on her left forearm. She explains that it has been there for the past two years and has gradually increased in size and she is embarrassed by its appearance. She explains that it feels as though the lesion is "stuck onto" the surface of her skin and it is almost as if she could just "pick it off" with her fingernail. On examination there is a solitary 15 mm diameter raised brown plaque like thickening on her left forearm with a waxy surface.
4. A 45-year-old woman attends your clinic with a rash in bilateral axillae and groins. She is a type 2 diabetic and has a history of PCOS. On examination there is a symmetrical, dark brown, velvety rash in the affected areas.
5. A 34-year-old woman presents to your clinic with multiple worsening depigmented areas on her trunk and limbs. She has a history of pernicious anaemia and had her last B12 injection three months ago. On examination there are several well defined milky white patches across her body.

See pages 53–54 for answers.

ANSWERS

Childhood infections 1

1. K. Scarlet fever
This is a bacterial illness caused by group A streptococcus. This patient has typical examination findings.

2. B. Erythema infectiosum
Also known as fifth disease, this condition is caused by parvovirus B19.

3. C. Hand, foot and mouth disease
This is a very infectious viral illness caused by the Coxsackie virus.

4. A. Chicken pox
This highly contagious condition results in an itchy, blistering rash and is caused by the varicella zoster virus.

5. F. Molluscum contagiosum
This is a contagious condition caused by the molluscum contagiosum virus.

6. H. Rheumatic fever
This patient has had a streptococcal infection recently and now presents with a combination of major and minor criteria for diagnosis of acute rheumatic fever.

Childhood infections 2

1. D. Kawasaki syndrome
This is an acute febrile illness in children which affects the small- and medium-sized blood vessels, particularly the coronary arteries.

2. E. Measles
This is a highly contagious condition caused by the measles virus. This was once a very widespread condition but in countries where measles is part of the vaccination schedule the incidence is very low.

3. I. Roseola infantum
This condition results from infection with human herpes virus 6. It is characterised by high fevers lasting between three to five days followed by rash development.

4. L. Staphylococcal scalded skin syndrome
This is a serious skin infection which develops as a result of a toxin produced by a staphylococcal infection.

5. G. Mumps
This condition is caused by an RNA paramyxovirus. Patients typically present with a prodrome of low-grade fever, myalgia, headaches and anorexia followed by swollen parotid glands.

Skin reactions

1. C. DRESS syndrome
This patient has had a severe drug reaction to lamotrigine, she also has eosinophilia and systemic symptoms. This condition usually appears two to eight weeks after starting an offending medication.

2. G. Porphyria cutanea tarda

This is the most common type of porphyria and is due to a defect in a liver enzyme called uroporphyrinogen decarboxylase (UROD). Urine samples demonstrate a characteristic coral coloured fluorescence when placed under Wood's lamp.

3. A. Acute generalised exanthematous pustulosis

Also known as toxic pustuloderma, this is an acute drug reaction which is characterised by development of pinhead sized, non-follicular pustules on erythematous skin. The rash usually lasts for about ten days and then resolves by peeling off.

4. F. Jarisch–Herxheimer reaction

This is a reaction which may be seen in individuals infected with spirochetes who commence treatment with antibiotics. It occurs within 24 hours of commencement of treatment.

5. E. Fixed drug eruption

This is an oval shaped erythematous lesion which develops after taking the offending drug. These usually recur at the same site after re-exposure to the same drug.

6. H. Stevens–Johnson syndrome

This is a life-threatening skin condition which requires prompt treatment. Sulfonamides are a common cause of this reaction.

Hair

1. E. Hypertrichosis

This condition involves excessive hair growth beyond what is normal for gender, age and race. It should not be confused with hirsutism which is hair growth in women which follows a male pattern of distribution.

2. A. Alopecia areata

This is an autoimmune condition which can lead to hair loss. The hair loss occurs in small patches. This patient has typical examination findings.

3. H. Telogen effluvium

This is a common cause of temporary hair loss due to excessive shedding of telogen hair. Acute episodes are commonly caused by a significant physical stressor.

4. J. Trichotillomania

This is a psychological disorder which involves an urge to pull at hair from various areas of the body.

5. D. Hirsutism

This condition involves male pattern hair growth which occurs in women. It should not be confused with hypertrichosis, a condition which involves excessive hair growth beyond what is normal for gender, age and race.

6. I. Tinea capitis

Also known as ringworm of the scalp, this is a rash which is caused by a fungal infection.

Nails 1

1. Q. Subungual hematoma

This results from bleeding under the nail and is usually secondary to trauma or repetitive micro trauma to the affected nail.

2. O. Panchyonychia congenita

This patient has typical examination findings including palmoplantar keratoderma and nail thickening.

3. P. Psoriasis

This patient has typical nail findings associated with psoriasis; the skin findings are also consistent with this diagnosis.

4. K. Myxoid cyst

These are benign growths which affect the digits but most commonly occur on the fingers.

5. B. Acute paronychia

This is a rapidly developing infection of the nail fold which is commonly associated with trauma.

Nails 2

1. N. Onycholysis

This is a common nail condition in which the nail separates from the nail bed giving a characteristic appearance in which the distal nail appears grayish-white in color.

2. D. Candida onychia

Diabetics and immunocompromised individuals are at greater risk of this condition.

3. M. Onychogryphosis

This is a condition more commonly seen in the elderly and usually results from poor footwear.

4. A. Acrolentiginous melanoma

This condition usually affects the thumb or great toe and is unrelated to sun exposure. Patients typically present with a narrow-pigmented band which widens and becomes more irregular. Hutchinson sign describes extension of the pigmentation to involve the skin of the nail fold.

5. E. Chronic paronychia

This condition is diagnosed clinically and is characterised by symptoms lasting greater than six weeks. Chronic paronychia results from irritant dermatitis.

Nail signs of systemic illness

1. A. Apparent leukonychia

This patient has Terry type nails which can be associated with hepatic disorders.

2. C. Koilonychia

This describes a thin spoon shaped nail, which is a common finding in iron deficiency anaemia.

3. B. Beau's lines

These are transverse depressions which result from disruption of nail growth. These are a common finding in patients undergoing chemotherapy.

4. D. Periungual fibroma

Also known as Koenen tumors, these are benign lesions affecting the nails of individuals with tuberous sclerosis.

5. H. Yellow nail syndrome

This is a nail condition in which there is a yellow discoloration of the nails and apparent growth cessation. It is commonly associated with pleural effusions and lymphoedema, the exact cause is unknown.

Dermatitis 1

1. H. Lichen simplex chronicus

This is a chronic form of dermatitis which results from repeated scratching of skin.

2. B. Asteatotic dermatitis

Also known as eczema craquele, this is a common form of dermatitis which occurs as a result of dry skin.

3. K. Seborrheic dermatitis

This is a skin condition which causes red patches and scaling, it typically affects areas with high sebum production.

4. A. Allergic contact dermatitis

This is a form of eczema which is caused by an allergic reaction as a result of an allergen coming into contact with the skin. This patient has likely been re-exposed to a substance to which they have been sensitised.

Dermatitis 2

1. F. Dyshidrotic eczematous dermatitis

Also known as vesicular hand dermatitis or pompholyx, this is a form of eczema characterised by vesicle or bullae formation.

2. C. Atopic dermatitis

This is the most common form of inflammatory skin disease in all patients. This is a chronic condition and patients have periodic flare-ups.

3. I. Nummular eczema

Also known as discoid eczema, this is a common form of eczema in which there are well defined scattered coin-shaped eczematous plaques.

4. G. Irritant contact dermatitis

This is a form of dermatitis which is localised to the area which has been exposed to the irritant. The hands are most commonly affected. Patients typically describe a burning, painful sensation rather than an itch as is seen in allergic contact dermatitis.

Inflammatory disorders 1

1. E. Granuloma annulare

This patient has presented with the localised form of granuloma annulare which is the most common type. These lesions typically present as flesh-coloured raised rings which typically form in the skin over joints.

2. M. Pyoderma gangrenosum

This condition presents with rapidly enlarging painful ulcers which result from a history of minor trauma. The ulcers have a characteristic purple border.

3. O. Sweet's syndrome

This patient has presented with neutrophilic dermatosis of the dorsal hands, this is a localised variant of sweet's syndrome. This patient demonstrates classical examination findings including pseudo-vesiculation.

4. H. Lichen planus

This is an autoimmune disorder which is mediated by T cells. The description of the lesions and their location support the diagnosis. The fine white lines represent Wickham striae.

Inflammatory disorders 2

1. K. Pityriasis rosea

The patient initially presented with a herald patch which is a pink to red coloured plaque with peripheral scaling within its edge. The secondary rash usually occurs two weeks after the herald patch first presents.

2. I. Morphea

This patient has presented with linear morphea which is the most common type found in children.

3. D. Erythema nodosum

This is an inflammatory condition which affects subcutaneous fat, they can be associated with streptococcal infections as illustrated in this case. This patient has classic examination findings.

4. C. Erythema multiforme

This is an immune mediated mucocutaneous condition which is usually self-limiting. Patients present with symmetrical distribution of target lesions which are pathognomonic for this condition. Most cases are precipitated by herpes simplex virus infections.

Skin lesions 1

1. K. Pilar cyst

Also known as a trichilemmal cyst these are keratin filled cysts which are most commonly found on the scalp. Unlike an epidermoid cyst they lack a central punctum and lack a granular layer on histology.

2. H. Keratoacanthoma

Also known as molluscum sebaceum, this is a rapidly growing skin lesion which is difficult to distinguish from a squamous cell carcinoma.

3. A. Actinic keratoses

These are pre-cancerous scaly lesions which occur secondary to sun damage.

4. B. Basal cell carcinoma

The correct answer is Basal cell carcinoma. Also known as a rodent ulcer, this is a common non-melanoma cancer.

5. D. Dermatofibroma

The correct answer is dermatofibroma. Also known as a cutaneous fibrous histiocytoma, these are benign nodules which are most commonly found in the lower limbs.

6. O. Squamous cell carcinoma in situ

The correct answer is Squamous cell carcinoma in situ. Also known as Bowen's disease, this is a slow growing skin cancer which appears as an erythematous, scaly plaque.

Skin lesions 2

1. M. Pyogenic granuloma

This condition is a benign proliferation of capillary blood vessels of the oral mucosa and skin.

2. G. Invasive squamous cell carcinoma

This is the second most common cause of skin cancer.

3. L. Polymorphous light eruption

This is a rash which is triggered by sun exposure. This patient has classic examination findings.

4. N. Solar lentigo

Also known as an old age spot, this is a benign skin lesion which occurs secondary to sun exposure.

5. C. Chondrodermatitis nodularis helicis

This is a tender cutaneous lesion which is commonly found over the helix of the ear. This patient presents with classic features and examination findings.

Pigmentation disorders 1

1. C. Erythrasma

This is a bacterial skin infection caused by the bacteria *Corynebacterium minutissimum*.

2. K. Poikiloderma of Civatte

This is a condition which is caused by sun exposure and results in skin discoloration and atrophy of sun exposed areas.

3. J. Pityriasis versicolor

This is a skin condition caused by Malassezia fungal growth.

4. P. Tuberous sclerosis

This is a multisystem genetic disease which can cause seizures, cognitive impairment and delayed development. Dermatological features include ash-leaf patches, shagreen patches and facial angiofibromas.

5. N. Tinea nigra

This is a mould infection, caused by *Hortaea werneckii*, which typically affects the palms or soles.

Pigmentation disorders 2

1. I. Pityriasis alba

This is a common eczematous rash in which individuals typically present with round or oval patches of hypopigmentation.

2. D. Melasma

Also known as the mask of pregnancy or chloasma, this is an acquired pigmentary disorder. Pregnancy is a factor which implicated in the development of this condition.

3. L. Seborrheic keratosis

This is a benign skin lesion which can arise anywhere on the skin surface except the palms and soles. They typically appear to be stuck onto the surface of the skin similar to barnacles.

4. A. Acanthosis nigricans

This is a skin condition in which patients present with dark discoloration which is typically found in the folds and creases.

5. Q. Vitiligo

This is considered an autoimmune condition in which the skin loses its pigmentation resulting in patches of depigmented skin.

Psychiatry

3

MOOD DISORDERS 1

A. Catatonia
B. Cyclothymic disorder
C. Bipolar I disorder
D. Bipolar II disorder
E. Brief psychotic disorder
F. Delusional disorder
G. Disruptive mood dysregulation disorder
H. Major depressive disorder
 I. Persistent depressive disorder (dysthymia)
J. Premenstrual dysphoric disorder
K. Schizophreniform disorder
L. Schizophrenia
M. Schizoaffective disorder – Bipolar type
N. Schizoaffective disorder – Depressive type

For each of the following, what is the MOST likely diagnosis?

1. A 10-year-old child presents to your clinic with his parents who can no longer cope with his behaviour. He has had regular tantrums on an almost daily basis for the past two years, his tantrums involve damaging items, yelling and physical aggression. Symptoms occur within the home, in public spaces and at school. His mother was particularly distressed about a recent episode where he lay in a shopping centre aisle crying when told he could not have a chocolate bar.

2. A 20-year-old presents with his concerned parents. He has been locking himself up in his room for most of the day and his mother has heard him speaking to other people when there is nobody present in the room with him. On questioning he reports that he does not leave the house as the police had placed cameras on his street six weeks ago to monitor where he goes. He had to take leave from his university course nine months ago as he was hospitalised with similar symptoms, his parents explain that he has gradually worsened since he was discharged.

3. A 32-year-old attends with her mother who explains that she has not been herself for the past six months. She will not leave the house and is worried that she is being followed. She believes that the Russian family who have moved in across the road from her house are spies and is reluctant to leave the home as she believes they are recording her movements. For the past week she has been talking a lot about her plans to create a charity to turn the Sahara Desert green, she has been spending a great deal of time on the internet researching her plans. She has had very poor sleep, averaging three to four hours a night but feeling refreshed after her sleep. Her mum has looked through her phone and has seen that she has been sending nude pictures of herself to random men.

4. An 18-year-old presents with her concerned parents. She has been behaving peculiarly for the past six weeks. She has been spending a great deal of time on the internet researching the FBI as she believes they have been tracking her. She has been hearing their voices through the bugs they have placed in her room; she has not been able to find these bugs as yet and her parents have not heard these noises. She has no significant past medical history.

See page 75 for answers.

MOOD DISORDERS 2

A. Catatonia
B. Cyclothymic disorder
C. Bipolar I disorder
D. Bipolar II disorder
E. Brief psychotic disorder
F. Delusional disorder
G. Disruptive mood dysregulation disorder
H. Major depressive disorder
I. Persistent depressive disorder (dysthymia)
J. Premenstrual dysphoric disorder
K. Schizophreniform disorder
L. Schizophrenia
M. Schizoaffective disorder – Bipolar type
N. Schizoaffective disorder – Depressive type

For each of the following, what is the MOST likely diagnosis?

1. A 55-year-old man presents with depressed mood for the past four months since the sudden passing of his wife in a motor vehicle accident. He has lost pleasure in all activities, has not been sleeping well and has lost 12 kg during this period of time. He is consumed by guilt over the passing of his wife, she was driving to

pick him up from work at the time. He has not had any suicidal ideations during this time.

2. A 65-year-old male has become over protective of his wife of 25 years and is at times aggressive towards her. He has seen her talking with the mail man a 21-year-old male and believes she has been having an affair with him for the past two months. He has followed her and has seen her posting letters in the local mail box, he believes these are meant for the mail man.

3. An 18-year-old has been having very severe mood swings associated with over-whelming fatigue. She gets very angry, feels on edge and feels as though she is out of control. She argues with her boyfriend more frequently, has been taking time off from university and she explains that she is desperate to find a solution for her presentation as she is very distressed. Her symptoms last for about five days and have been happening almost every month a few days before onset of menses and improve shortly after this.

4. A 36-year-old recently had a falling out with his fiancée, he reports that he has not been able to function properly for the past three weeks. He has been in bed for most of the day during this period of time, has been feeling very hopeless and worthless. He has been eating poorly and has gained 8 kg during this time. He has not attended work as he cannot focus on his duties, his employer has asked him to take time off to get his affairs in order. He explains that he has not been like this before. Three months ago, he was able to go to work, tutor after work and write a book while sleeping only four hours a night. Despite the lack of sleep, he felt well rested.

5. A 32-year-old presents with her parents who tell you she has been behaving in a peculiar manner for the past two weeks. She has been posting on social media about her plans to end poverty in Central Africa, her posts are made at odd hours of the night and day. On review she is very talkative and explains that she is full of energy, she tells you she has been sleeping for about three to four hours a night and feels well rested. Her mother tells you she has also been sending sexually explicit text messages to her male colleagues. She has no past medical history and a urine drug test is negative.

See page 75 for answers.

SLEEP DISTURBANCES 1

A. **Adjustment sleep disorder**
B. **Kleine–Levin syndrome**
C. **Caffeine induced sleep disorder**
D. **Central sleep apnoea**
E. **Narcolepsy**
F. **Obstructive sleep apnoea**

G. **Periodic limb movement disorder**
H. **REM sleep behaviour disorder**
 I. **Restless leg syndrome**
 J. **Sleep offset insomnia**
K. **Sleep terror**
L. **Somnambulism**

For each of the following, what is the MOST likely diagnosis?

1. A 39-year-old woman presents with wrist pain, she reports that she had a dream that she was being attacked by a dog and struck out at the dog. She was awoken by her husband whom she had been punching in her sleep. Her husband reports that she has had several episodes like this and that on waking her up she is oriented and alert. He reports that the symptoms happen about two hours into sleep and he is now fearful of sleeping near her. She is deeply distressed by the impact of her behaviour.

2. A 28-year-old presents with recurrent episodes of irrepressible need to sleep and daytime napping. Her symptoms happen on most days of the week and have been going on for the past four months. Nocturnal sleep polysomnography is arranged which reveals REM sleep latency of 13 minutes.

3. A 5-year-old girl has had recurrent episodes of waking in the middle of the night. She screams and is significantly distressed during the episodes and her mother struggles to comfort her. She can't remember the episodes in the morning.

4. A 51-year-old man attends with his wife who complains that he moves his legs at night and it is keeping her awake. She explains that it usually happens a couple of hours after they go to bed. He reports that he has no recollection of these movements, he does however report that his sleep is disturbed and he is drowsy during the day. You arrange a sleep study for him which reveals episodes of leg movements at least 20 times per hour.

See pages 75–76 for answers.

SLEEP DISTURBANCES 2

A. **Adjustment sleep disorder**
B. **Kleine–Levin syndrome**
C. **Caffeine induced sleep disorder**
D. **Central sleep apnoea**
E. **Narcolepsy**
 F. **Obstructive sleep apnoea**
G. **Periodic limb movement disorder**
H. **REM sleep behaviour disorder**

I. Restless leg syndrome
J. Sleep offset insomnia
K. Sleep terror
L. Somnambulism

For each of the following, what is the MOST likely diagnosis?

1. A 23-year-old presents with sleep disturbance. For the past two weeks he has struggled to sleep and has remained awake for most of the night. He gets between four and five hours of sleep a night as a result of his symptoms. He has been very stressed as he has recently been promoted at work and has been struggling with the additional work load.

2. A 54-year-old truck driver presents to your clinic complaining of fatigue. He explains that he is tired throughout the day and has had a few incidents at work where he has fallen asleep briefly at the wheel of his vehicle. He has a poor sleep and is restless throughout, causing his wife to wake up several times during the night. On examination he has a BMI of 38, blood pressure of 158/92 mmHg, respiratory rate of 18 and a heart rate of 86 beats per minute.

3. A 35-year-old man attends your clinic with his partner who explains that she has found him in the kitchen in the middle of the night on several occasions during the past six months. When she approaches him during these episodes, he has a blank stare and is unresponsive. In the morning he has no recollection of the events and reports that he has no memory of any dreams.

4. A 21-year-old presents with insomnia for the past six months, He reports it has been hard for him to initiate and maintain sleep. He reports that he is particularly bothered by an urge to move his legs at night, he has to get up to walk about his room to relieve his symptoms and it is affecting his relationship with his girlfriend as he occasionally kicks her at night. He has a history of iron deficiency and takes iron supplements when he can. He reports that he is otherwise well.

See page 76 for answers.

ANXIETY 1

A. Acute stress disorder
B. Adjustment disorder
C. Agoraphobia
D. Body dysmorphic disorder
E. Dermatillomania
F. Ekbom's syndrome
G. Generalised anxiety disorder
H. Hoarding disorder

I. Obsessive compulsive disorder
J. Panic attack
K. Panic disorder
L. Post-Traumatic stress disorder (PTSD)
M. Selective mutism
N. Separation anxiety disorder
O. Social anxiety disorder
P. Specific phobia

For each of the following, what is the MOST likely diagnosis?

1. A 7-year-old girl takes plenty of sick leave from school. When her parents try to take her to school, she complains of stomach pain and headaches. She clings on to her mother when she is taken to school and her teachers have to physically remove her from her mother.
2. A 21-year-old has recently commenced a job with a public relations firm. He was initially very excited about his job but now struggles with his role. He dislikes chairing meetings and public speaking; he feels as though his peers are judging him and that he will make a mistake that will embarrass him in front of them.
3. A 23-year-old had a horse-riding accident two weeks ago; her horse was put down as a result of the accident and she sustained a broken arm. She has flash backs to the event and nightmares.
4. A 38-year-old soldier was stationed in Iraq for three years, during his time there he witnessed a suicide bombing in a busy market place which took the life of a colleague and dozens of civilians. The event took place one year ago but he relives the event almost daily, he has ongoing nightmares, poor sleep and suffers from anxiety as a result. He avoids market places.
5. A 42-year-old is deeply concerned about everything and constantly feels as though bad things are about to happen. She explains that her symptoms have become significantly worse over the past year and reports that it is affecting her sleep, she is tired on most days and always feels tense.

See page 76 for answers.

ANXIETY 2

A. Acute stress disorder
B. Adjustment disorder
C. Agoraphobia
D. Body dysmorphic disorder
E. Dermatillomania
F. Ekbom's syndrome
G. Generalised anxiety disorder

H. Hoarding disorder
I. Obsessive compulsive disorder
J. Panic attack
K. Panic disorder
L. Post-Traumatic stress disorder (PTSD)
M. Selective mutism
N. Separation anxiety disorder
O. Social anxiety disorder
P. Specific phobia

For each of the following, what is the MOST likely diagnosis?

1. A 56-year-old presents with rectal bleeding and loss of weight, he was sent for a colonoscope which he had two days ago. The colonoscope reveals that he has evidence of bowel cancer. Since hearing this news, he has been very low and teary.

2. A 22-year-old woman presents with worsening anxiety. She is a university student and has been struggling to attend her classes. She finds the lecture halls large and overwhelming, and has found that over the past few months she has slowly withdrawn from in person sessions to now watching her lectures online from home.

3. A 22-year-old woman was out with her friends. She explains that she suddenly noticed her heart begin to race, she felt tightness in her chest and reports that she felt short of breath. She presents at your emergency department where you review her. You find no abnormality on physical examination or investigation.

4. A 28-year-old presents with severe dermatitis in both hands, on questioning he reports a three-year history of repetitive hand washing. He explains that he always feels as though his hands are contaminated with germs. His thoughts cause him much distress but he cannot resist the urge to wash his hands.

5. An 18-year-old presents with a recent history of weight loss, 6 kg in the past month. On questioning she is overly concerned about her body size.

6. A 22-year-old presents with a small lesion on her right wrist which has become infected. You ask her to remove her jumper so that you can assess the lesion properly and note that she has many similar lesions extending up to her elbow. You review her notes and see that she has attended the clinic many times in the past with similar presentations. She reluctantly admits that she picks at her skin when she is anxious and has sought help in the past to try and stop this behaviour.

See page 77 for answers.

BEHAVIOURAL CONDITIONS 1

A. Antisocial personality disorder
B. Attention deficit hyperactivity disorder (ADHD)
C. Autism spectrum disorder

D. Borderline personality disorder
E. Conduct disorder
F. Intermittent explosive disorder
G. Kleptomania
H. Malingering
 I. Oppositional defiant disorder
J. Pyromania

For each of the following, what is the MOST likely diagnosis?

1. A 12-year-old school boy often gets into trouble at school. He is disorganised and forgetful, he does not complete his homework and struggles to focus in class.
2. A 21-year-old woman presents with her partner who is concerned that she criticises herself excessively and lacks clear goals in her life. He explains that she spends a lot of time online in chat groups and social media and that she lashes out at anybody that criticises her online. He tells you that on a few occasions her anger has been so extreme that she contacted individuals she knew offline to vent at them as soon as they had posted their criticisms, she cares little about the consequences of her actions. He is concerned as during her episodes she spends in anger and exceeds their budget without regard. She also gets into her car when angry and drives recklessly and has had many near misses. Her partner has been struggling with her behaviours and has threatened to leave the relationship but she has done everything she can to try and keep them together. She has recurrently threatened self-harm to achieve her goals.
3. A 29-year-old doctor has been working in a metropolitan hospital for the past 12 months. She loses her temper often with junior medical and nursing staff, she is described by her colleagues as often angry and resentful, interns feel as though she blames them for her mistakes. Senior medical staff within her unit complain that she is argumentative and is known to refuse reasonable requests. She deliberately creates unnecessary tasks for nursing staff and junior doctors she dislikes.
4. A 21-year-old presents to your emergency department under police escort. He has been involved in an altercation and has sustained multiple small injuries. He is irritable on review and explains that he "smashed the guy at the pub really good" because "he looked at me funny, he deserves what he got". You review his hospital file and see that he has attended the department for similar such presentations since the age of 13. The police officers explain that he is well known to them.

See page 77 for answers.

BEHAVIOURAL CONDITIONS 2

A. Antisocial personality disorder
B. Attention deficit hyperactivity disorder (ADHD)

C. Autism spectrum disorder
D. Borderline personality disorder
E. Conduct disorder
F. Intermittent explosive disorder
G. Kleptomania
H. Malingering
 I. Oppositional defiant disorder
J. Pyromania

For each of the following, what is the MOST likely diagnosis?

1. A 16-year-old boy attends the clinic with his mother. He has attended for review of his right hand which is swollen as a result of a playground fight for which he was suspended from school. He has a history of marijuana use and has been arrested multiple times in the past three years for drug and weapon possession, destruction of public property and physical violence against others. He was recently released from juvenile detention after spending some time there for burning down a house.

2. A 42-year-old man started stealing from the age of twenty-two, he has been arrested several times for this but has continued to do so. He explains that he does not need the small objects he steals but cannot resist the urge to steal them. He derives great satisfaction from these acts and discards the items shortly after the offences are committed.

3. A 14-year-old girl presents with her mother who is concerned about her behaviour at school. She insists on the same routine at school and becomes very distressed if teachers are away or classes are changed. When things change, she refuses to follow teacher instructions and lashes out at staff. She does not have any friends at school and does not attempt to play with any other children. She enjoys mathematics at school and has been doing very well in this subject but is significantly behind her peers in other subjects.

4. An unemployed 24-year-old male presents requesting a letter of support, he was recently arrested by police for possession of stolen goods. He has been robbing homes in his local neighbourhood and selling the goods online. He explains that he believes he is suffering from a psychiatric condition, he explains that he has been stealing since he was a child and he does not know why he does it. His lawyer has asked him to present to you for a letter as it may help his court case.

See pages 77–78 for answers.

MEMORY 1

A. Alzheimer's dementia
B. Creutzfeldt–Jakob disease

C. **Frontotemporal dementia**
D. **HIV associated dementia**
E. **Huntington's disease**
F. **Korsakoff syndrome**
G. **Lewy body dementia**
H. **Normal pressure hydrocephalus**
 I. **Parkinson's disease**
J. **Pseudodementia**
K. **Neurosyphilis**
L. **Vascular dementia**
M. **Wernicke's encephalopathy**

For each of the following, what is the MOST likely diagnosis?

1. A 56-year-old woman presents with her daughter who tells you that she does not seem to be the same person, her daughter explains that she is very withdrawn. Examination reveals that she cannot name a pen or a watch or explain their function but you find no concerning features with regard to her short-term memory.

2. A 78-year-old has been suffering from memory loss for the past six months. During this time, she has had several falls, her most recent fall last week has ended her up in hospital with a significant laceration to the right side of her head requiring sutures. She has a history significant for hypertension and hyperlipidaemia. On examination she has a broad-based gait with outward rotated feet. You perform an MMSE and she scores 18/30. Her daughter adds that she has been having issues controlling her urine and has had a lot of accidents in the past six months.

3. A 66-year-old smoker presents with a three-month history memory loss, speech difficulty, unsteady gait and difficulty swallowing. His symptoms began after a stroke but have been worsening in a step wise manner. He has a past medical history significant for hypertension, hyperlipidaemia and type 2 diabetes mellitus. His current medications include captopril, atorvastatin and metformin. Examination reveals asymmetric reflexes and speech difficulty.

4. A 46-year-old presents to your emergency department with police. He was found on a bench in a public park in a confused state, police try to get him up to walk but he cannot lift himself and is unable to walk even with the support of the officers. He cannot recall how he got there and cannot recall his address or who his next of kin is. On examination he has a heart rate of 68 bpm, temp 36.7°C and BP of 118/90 mmHg. You note bruising across his body, clubbing of his fingers, palmar erythema, decreased body hair and mild gynaecomastia. Abdominal examination reveals an enlarged liver, he also has nystagmus with bilateral lateral recti palsy.

See page 78 for answers.

MEMORY 2

A. Alzheimer's dementia
B. Creutzfeldt–Jakob disease
C. Frontotemporal dementia
D. HIV associated dementia
E. Huntington's disease
F. Korsakoff syndrome
G. Lewy body dementia
H. Normal pressure hydrocephalus
 I. Parkinson's disease
 J. Pseudodementia
K. Neurosyphilis
L. Vascular dementia
M. Wernicke's encephalopathy

For each of the following, what is the MOST likely diagnosis?

1. A 58-year-old male presents with a two-year history of worsening memory loss, poor concentration, anxiety and agitation. He has been suffering from episodes of vertigo, tinnitus and hearing loss during this time. He also reports episodes of sudden excruciating eye pain which has caused his eyes to tear up and is associated with photosensitivity. He reports that he feels weaker by the day, has burning sensations in his hands and toes, decreased sense of touch in these areas and has been struggling with urinary incontinence. On examination he walks in a jerky, non-fluid manner, pupils are equal but have an impaired response to light, diminished deep tendon reflexes with an absent knee jerk.

2. A 64-year-old male presents to your clinic after having had a fall at home. He has had two other falls in the past six months. On presentation he is able to ambulate, but you note that he does so with a shuffling motion. His son reports that he has become increasingly forgetful, yesterday he came over to his house to check on him and found that he had left the stove on for too long and burnt his dinner. His son explains that he has been forgetting to attend his appointments and family events. On examination, there is pronounced bradykinesia in his upper limbs associated with cogwheel rigidity. You review his past history and note that he has had this stiffness for some time and was prescribed medication to treat this 13 months ago.

3. A 48-year-old man attends your clinic with his wife, who tells you she is concerned about his change in personality in recent times. Over the past six months he has been very impulsive and irritable. He has been very forgetful during this time, has been missing work and not turning up to events at his daughter's school. She has noticed that he has also had very fast jerking movements at times and twitching in his face and arms. His father and uncle had dementia in their 50s but the family are unsure of what the exact cause was as it happened

overseas before they migrated to this country. You arrange for a CT scan of his brain which reveals atrophic changes in the caudate nuclei.

4. An 88-year-old veteran has been brought into your emergency department for review by his concerned daughter who complains that her father has become increasingly confused and that his memory is worsening. He was seen by your colleague and you note in his file that his last MMSE was 16/30. His daughter is however concerned about his more recent symptoms, over the past week she has found him wandering about the house, on questioning he has explained to her that he was following "the little men" within their hallway. He has not been unwell and has had no fevers, he is comfortable and without pain or injury. You perform a urine dipstick which is clear and he has an expressionless face.

See pages 78–79 for answers.

PARAPHILIC CONDITIONS 1

A. Exhibitionistic disorder
B. Fetishistic disorder
C. Frotteuristic disorder
D. Paedophilic disorder – exclusive type
E. Paedophilic disorder – non-exclusive type
F. Sexual masochism disorder
G. Sexual sadism disorder
H. Transvestic disorder with autogynephilia
 I. Transvestic disorder with fetishism
J. Voyeuristic disorder

For each of the following, what is the MOST likely diagnosis?

1. A 56-year-old is concerned about a skin lesion on her neck. On examination the lesion appears benign but you note bruising around her neck. You are concerned for her safety and question her about the bruise marks. She reluctantly opens up to you and explains that she has been engaging in new sexual practices. She reports that she derives pleasure from being humiliated and afflicted with pain by her partner. She explains that she also participates in activities involving the restriction of breathing, this is what has caused the bruising on her neck.

2. A 29-year-old office worker attends your clinic as he is very distressed. For the past year he has secretly been purchasing women's high heel shoes online. He explains that he is obsessed with shoes and feet in particular, he has intense sexual arousal as a result of his obsession. At work he cannot focus, he is constantly looking at the shoes and feet of his female co-workers and reports that it is causing him much distress.

3. A 16-year-old boy has been fantasising about a young girl who comes on his school bus, she started at the school nine months ago and he cannot get her out of his thoughts. He has intense sexual fantasies about her but has never acted on them. He is really distressed by his feeling and would like help as they are now beginning to impact his daily functions. The girl is 9-years-old. He has never had any sexual interests in the past.
4. A 26-year-old explains that he enjoys thinking about cross dressing. He tells you that he is extremely obsessed with women's clothing and fabrics more than anything else and he derives intense sexual pleasure from his feelings.

See page 79 for answers.

PARAPHILIC CONDITIONS 2

A. **Exhibitionistic disorder**
B. **Fetishistic disorder**
C. **Frotteuristic disorder**
D. **Paedophilic disorder – exclusive type**
E. **Paedophilic disorder – non-exclusive type**
F. **Sexual masochism disorder**
G. **Sexual sadism disorder**
H. **Transvestic disorder with autogynephilia**
I. **Transvestic disorder with fetishism**
J. **Voyeuristic disorder**

For each of the following, what is the MOST likely diagnosis?

1. A 36-year-old requests a letter of support for an upcoming court case. He has been attending large music events where has been rubbing his genitals against women in the crowd. He has attended multiple events in the past 12 months and has been removed from several of these by security for his behaviour. He reports that he gets intense sexual arousal from doing this.
2. A 56-year-old has been arrested by police after being found in the backyard of a house at night performing a sexual act on himself. He was looking through the blinds of a bedroom where an 18-year-old school girl had been undressing. She heard a noise outside her window and contacted police. He has been arrested for similar behaviour multiple times over the past five years.
3. You are called by the local police department to see a 38-year-old male who has sustained some injuries while being arrested by the police. He was arrested for domestic violence. On examination he has some minor cuts on his hands that do not need treatment. On questioning he explains that he has been emotionally and psychologically abusive towards his partner for several years and over the

past six months has progressively become more physically violent. He explains that he derives intense sexual pleasure from seeing his partner suffer.

4. A 32-year-old has been exposing his genitals to primary school girls walking home from school and to women jogging on a footpath near his home. He has been doing this for the past ten months and has recently been arrested for this behaviour after being found by police outside of a primary school. He explains that he gets intense sexual arousal as a result of exposing himself to these individuals.

See pages 79–80 for answers.

PERSONALITY DISORDERS 1

A. Antisocial personality disorder
B. Avoidant personality disorder
C. Borderline personality disorder
D. Dependent personality disorder
E. Histrionic personality disorder
 F. Narcissistic personality disorder
G. Obsessive compulsive personality disorder
H. Paranoid personality disorder
 I. Schizoid personality disorder
 J. Schizotypal personality disorder

For each of the following, what is the MOST likely diagnosis?

1. A 36-year-old GP, who works at your clinic, is worried that his patients will write negative reviews about him in online forums. He feels as though they make fun of him behind his back. He left his last practice as he did not get along with other doctors there, he believes that they had been ruining his name in the local community he has worked in.

2. A 21-year-old woman has recently commenced a job in an office. She feels like she would like to leave her job after two weeks as she feels awkward around her work colleagues, they are nice to her but she feels they see her as "odd and kind of weird". She stays at her desk during lunch breaks and does not go to the staff cafeteria as she feels very anxious around her colleagues and gets very embarrassed when they speak to her.

3. A 25-year-old woman attends your clinic complaining of back pain. She has come to see you for minor complaints in the past and has been very flirtatious during visits. Today she is upset at you as you have not made any comments about how her hair and clothing look, "doctor I am so hurt, I try to appear very nice when I come to see you". When you leave your office, you see her in the car park arguing with someone on the phone in a very loud voice, she is sitting at the kerbside and is extremely teary and emotional.

4. A 62-year-old lives at home alone with multiple cats. Her house is very cramped, run down and almost unliveable. She wears oddly paired old clothing that she has picked up from charity collection bins. Her daughter is concerned about her as she says very strange things, last week she threw out her television as she believed that the news bulletins were secretly sending out messages to the community about her. She has multiple rings with quartz crystals embedded in them which she tells you provides her protection against the evil of the world.

See page 80 for answers.

PERSONALITY DISORDERS 2

A. **Antisocial personality disorder**
B. **Avoidant personality disorder**
C. **Borderline personality disorder**
D. **Dependent personality disorder**
E. **Histrionic personality disorder**
F. **Narcissistic personality disorder**
G. **Obsessive compulsive personality disorder**
H. **Paranoid personality disorder**
I. **Schizoid personality disorder**
J. **Schizotypal personality disorder**

For each of the following, what is the MOST likely diagnosis?

1. A 32-year-old presents complaining that her life has fallen apart since her husband divorced her. She explains that she has lost her ability to function since this happened, has not been able to sleep and has a reduced appetite. She reports that she has no guidance as her ex-husband would normally make decisions for her. Her previous boyfriend is in attendance and tells you that she has been spending a lot of time at his house and sleeping over since her divorce. She explains that she is afraid to be alone and does not feel she can care for herself.

2. An unemployed 21-year-old man attends your ED after an altercation he had with an individual on the street, "he deserved what he got". He is well known to your department and has a long history of similar such presentations since he was at least 13. He has been arrested for assault on several occasions and is usually very aggressive with hospital staff.

3. A 26-year-old IT professional lives with her mother on an acreage but spends a great deal of time in her room alone, leaving her room only to use the bathroom or eat food. She works from home and enjoys her work as she spends a great deal of time alone. She has friends online with whom she plays online games but they have never met in person and only play every few months.

4. A 28-year-old surgical trainee attends your study group and praises her surgical skills excessively, she tells you about how she feels she is better than some of the more experienced surgeons. She does not seem to understand that others do not share the same view as her regarding her skills and tire from hearing herself praise. She was recently called into a meeting with her training supervisor as there were concerns about her ability to tie basic surgical knots. She gets very angry and accuses her supervisor of jealousy and tells him that he "can only wish" to be as good as her.

See page 80 for answers.

SUBSTANCE RELATED AND ADDICTIVE DISORDERS 1

A. Alcohol intoxication
B. Alcohol use disorder
C. Alcohol withdrawal
D. Amphetamine intoxication
E. Amphetamine withdrawal
F. Caffeine intoxication
G. Caffeine withdrawal
H. Cannabis intoxication
I. Cannabis use disorder
J. Cannabis withdrawal
K. Cocaine intoxication
L. Cocaine withdrawal
M. Opioid intoxication
N. Opioid use disorder
O. Opioid withdrawal
P. Phencyclidine intoxication
Q. Phencyclidine use disorder
R. Tobacco use disorder

For each of the following, what is the MOST likely diagnosis?

1. A 22-year-old woman has been found in a toilet cubicle at a night club by security guards in an agitated and anxious state. She is combative and tries to fight with the guards. Genia tells paramedics on arrival that she has chest pain. On examination she is diaphoretic, has a heart rate of 122 bpm, temp 36.3°C and BP of 172/102 mmHg. She has dilated pupils and evidence of nasal septum perforation. An ECG reveals ST elevation in leads II, III and aVF.

2. A 21-year-old university student is found by police sitting on the side of the road with his car keys on the floor beside him. His car is parked half on the curb and half on the road. Local members contacted police as they were concerned about an individual driving erratically through a shopping centre car park. He has slurred speech and is very aggressive with the police officers. He cannot walk to the police car as he is unsteady.

3. An 18-year-old university student is brought into hospital by ambulance. He was at a house party with friends and broke into a neighbour's house, screaming "people are after me" as he desperately tried to hide in a closet within their home. The neighbours called police and he was transferred to hospital. He has nil significant medical history. On examination he is appears very anxious, has a heart rate of 118 bpm, temp 36.8°C and BP of 116/84 mmHg. You observe conjunctival injection and dry mucous membranes. He asks for something to eat as he is very hungry.

4. A 28-year-old male is brought into the local emergency department under police escort. He was found outside a night club abusing members of the public. On examination he has a heart rate of 114 bpm, temp 36.2°C and BP of 157/100 mmHg. You note an ataxic gait, horizontal nystagmus and muscle rigidity.

5. A 52-year-old librarian attends your clinic for review. She has been very anxious and stressed over the past two days, she divorced her partner six months ago and feels as though things have gotten out of control. Her credit cards were cancelled a few days ago as she has not been keeping up with her payments. She tells you that she has not slept very well over the past few days. On examination she is diaphoretic, has a heart rate of 112 bpm, temp 37.1°C and BP of 132/86 mmHg.

See pages 80–81 for answers.

SUBSTANCE RELATED AND ADDICTIVE DISORDERS 2

A. **Alcohol intoxication**
B. **Alcohol use disorder**
C. **Alcohol withdrawal**
D. **Amphetamine intoxication**
E. **Amphetamine withdrawal**
F. **Caffeine intoxication**
G. **Caffeine withdrawal**
H. **Cannabis intoxication**
I. **Cannabis use disorder**
J. **Cannabis withdrawal**

   K. Cocaine intoxication
   L. Cocaine withdrawal
   M. Opioid intoxication
   N. Opioid use disorder
   O. Opioid withdrawal
   P. Phencyclidine intoxication
   Q. Phencyclidine use disorder
   R. Tobacco use disorder

For each of the following, what is the MOST likely diagnosis?

   1. A 22-year-old woman attends your ED with her parents who are concerned for her wellbeing. Fiona had an appendicectomy a few days ago and has been unable to leave her home. She has been very restless and anxious over the past four hours and her parents explain that she has had ongoing diarrhoea and vomiting during this period of time. On examination her pupils are dilated, she has a runny nose, a heart rate of 104 bpm, temp 36.2°C and BP of 128/80 mmHg.

   2. A 27-year-old male is brought to your emergency department after being found unresponsive at a house party. On arrival he is responsive only to painful stimuli, taking very shallow breaths and is cyanotic with pin point pupils. On examination he has a respiratory rate of five breaths/minute, heart rate of 64 bpm, temp 36.3°C and BP of 100/82 mmHg. You examine his chest and note crackles throughout his lungs.

   3. A 26-year-old gym enthusiast presents to his local emergency department. He tried a homemade high energy protein shake that his friend gave him for breakfast this morning then headed to the gym. Since completing his session, he has been very restless, nervous and has noticed that muscles in his arms and legs have been twitching. He has nil significant past medical history and takes no regular medication, he recently stopped drinking coffee as he was drinking six cups a day which was affecting his sleep. On examination he is very fidgety and has a flushed face, has a heart rate of 124 bpm, temp 36.8°C and BP of 122/78 mmHg. He collapses while you are reviewing him, an ECG reveals that he has gone into ventricular fibrillation. Despite your efforts he cannot be resuscitated.

   4. A 23-year-old journalist is brought to your clinic by her concerned parents. She has been behaving in an odd manner this morning, she has been very fidgety and extremely talkative. Her parents tell you that she has not been eating much over the past few days and has been awake for long periods of time at night writing a book. She tells you that she is "so full of energy" and reports she has been getting a lot done as she is very much focused. On examination she has a heart rate of 118 bpm, temp 37.8°C, RR 22 and BP of 154/98 mmHg. Her oral mucosa is dry and she has dilated pupils.

See page 81 for answers.

EATING DISORDERS 1

A. Anorexia nervosa
B. Avoidant restrictive food intake disorder
C. Binge eating disorder
D. Bulimia nervosa
E. Kleine–Levin syndrome
F. Night eating syndrome
G. Orthorexia nervosa
H. Pica
I. Purging disorder
J. Rumination disorder

For each of the following, what is the MOST likely diagnosis?

1. A 13-year-old girl presents with a significant amount of weight loss over the past 12 months and her family are worried about her wellbeing. She explains that she is not concerned about her body image or weight gain, rather she is afraid to eat. As she develops abdominal discomfort and nausea when she does. She has no medical history of concern and on examination she has a BMI of 14.6.

2. A 32-year-old pregnant woman is 38 weeks' gestation; she has had an uncomplicated pregnancy. For the past five weeks she has had an overwhelming urge to eat ice cubes, she has been freezing large quantities at home and her husband is concerned about her behaviour.

3. For the past six months a 19-year-old man has been eating small amounts of food during the day and he is concerned about this. He tells you that he spends a great deal of time awake at night as he has difficulty sleeping, during the night he eats significant quantities of food but does not feel unwell or uncomfortable as a result of what he consumes. He also wakes during the night to eat food even when he has had a reasonable dinner earlier in the night. He is drowsy during the day because of his eating habits.

4. A 23-year-old woman presents with abdominal discomfort and bloating. She explains that she has been having episodes where she eats excessive amounts of food for at least four to five days a month for the past 12 months and she tells you that she feels out of control with her food intake. She tells you that during episodes she eats alone as she is embarrassed by her behaviour, she eats very quickly and feels uncomfortably full when she is done. On examination she has a temp of 36.9°C, BP of 122/74 mmHg, HR 72, RR 20 and a BMI of 25.2. Abdominal examination reveals mild distension but is otherwise soft and non-tender. She is very distressed about her eating habits.

See pages 81–82 for answers.

EATING DISORDERS 2

A. Anorexia nervosa
B. Avoidant restrictive food intake disorder
C. Binge eating disorder
D. Bulimia nervosa
E. Kleine–Levin syndrome
F. Night eating syndrome
G. Orthorexia nervosa
H. Pica
I. Purging disorder
J. Rumination disorder

For each of the following, what is the MOST likely diagnosis?

1. A 25-year-old student attends with a long history of episodic periods of prolonged sleep. He sleeps up to 20 hours a day during episodes, he tells you that he has also had a significantly increased appetite and an abnormally increased sex drive.

2. A 21-year-old woman attends complaining of nausea and dizziness. She explains that she has been exercising for four hours a day for the past two weeks as she feels she has put on too much weight and she is depressed about this. She has been having episodes where she eats excessive amounts of food for about two days a week for the past six months and she tells you that she feels out of control with her food intake. On examination she has a temp of 36.6°C, BP of 98/68 mmHg, HR 62, RR 16 and a BMI of 19.2. You notice that the enamel of her anterior teeth is badly eroded.

3. A 26-year-old IT professional spends three to four hours during the day planning his diet, he explains to you that he is annoyed by his colleagues and partner who do not adhere to the same eating practices as himself, given that his diet is "by far better and healthier than theirs". He does not eat with his friends or family during special events like birthdays or Christmas as he does not wish to change his routine and clean eating is more important to him than these events. His behaviours are causing him to argue with his family, friends and partner.

4. A 17-year-old girl presents with a complaint of lethargy. On examination she has a BP of 80/62 mmHg, HR 42 and a BMI of 14.1. She attends with her grandmother who explains that she has lost 10 kg in the past two months, she exercises for at least two hours a day and has restricted her diet dramatically. Despite her low BMI she still believes she is overweight and expresses intense fear of weight gain.

See page 82 for answers.

ANSWERS

Mood disorders 1

1. G. Disruptive mood dysregulation disorder

This patient has severe recurrent temper outbursts that are out of proportion to the situation or provocation and inconsistent with his developmental level. His symptoms occur on a daily basis, have been present for at least 12 months and started before the age of 10.

2. L. Schizophrenia

This patient has a poor level of functioning, delusions and hallucinations lasting for at least six months without depression or mania.

3. M. Schizoaffective disorder – Bipolar type

She has an uninterrupted period of illness during which she has a manic episode. She has had delusions for more than two weeks in the absence of the manic episode.

4. K. Schizophreniform disorder

This patient has delusions and hallucinations lasting for at least one month but less than six months without depression or mania.

Mood disorders 2

1. H. Major depressive disorder

He has a depressed mood and loss of pleasure in activities. His symptoms have been present for over two weeks in duration.

2. F. Delusional disorder

He has had delusions present for one month or longer without meeting criteria A for schizophrenia. This presentation is an example of the jealous subtype of delusional disorder.

3. J. Premenstrual dysphoric disorder

This patient has at least five symptoms in the week prior to menses as outlined in the DSM 5. The patient is distressed by her symptoms and it is having an impact on her studies and relationship.

4. D. Bipolar II disorder

He has met the criteria for a major depressive disorder and at least one hypomanic episode.

5. C. Bipolar I disorder

She has met the criteria for at least one manic episode lasting at least one week in duration.

Sleep disturbances 1

1. H. REM sleep behaviour disorder

This patient has repeated episodes of arousal associated with reflex motor responses to the content of her dreams (dream enacting behaviour).

2. E. Narcolepsy

This patient has recurrent episodes of irrepressible need to sleep and day time napping occurring at least three times a week over a period of more than three months. She also has a REM sleep latency of less than or equal to 15 minutes.

3. K. Sleep terror

This is a form of non-REM sleep arousal disorder. This patient has recurrent episodes of abrupt terror arousals from sleep and no recollection of the events.

4. G. Periodic limb movement disorder

This involves involuntary limb movements during sleep which may result in poor quality sleep. Diagnosis requires greater than 15 periodic limb movements per hour in adults and more than five per hour in children.

Sleep disturbances 2

1. A. Adjustment sleep disorder

Also known as acute insomnia, this occurs as a result of acute stressors. The symptoms usually resolve when stressors are no longer present.

2. F. Obstructive sleep apnoea

This is a sleep disorder in which individuals have recurrent episodes of apnoea while asleep. This condition results in daytime sleepiness. This patient has several risk factors including obesity, male gender and hypertension.

3. L. Somnambulism

This is a form of non-REM sleep arousal disorder. This patient has recurrent episodes of sleep walking and no recollection of the events.

4. I. Restless leg syndrome

Also known as Willis–Ekbom disease, this condition involves a patient having an urge to move their lower limbs and relief by doing so. The symptoms usually come about while at rest and can result in insomnia. Iron deficiency is a common associated factor.

Anxiety 1

1. N. Separation anxiety disorder

The correct answer is separation anxiety disorder. This occurs when a child has intense worry and fear about parting from loved ones.

2. O. Social anxiety disorder

Patients with this condition experience fear, avoidance and anxiety in social settings. They typically report fear of being watched or judged by those around them.

3. A. Acute stress disorder

This condition differs to PTSD in the fact that the patient suffers from symptoms for three days to one month post the traumatic event.

4. L. Post-Traumatic stress disorder

He was exposed to a life-threatening traumatic event; he has recurrent distressing memories of the event and has been trying to avoid stimuli associated with the event. His symptoms have persisted for greater than one month

5. G. Generalised anxiety disorder

People with this condition worry uncontrollably about events and threats that may impact themselves or their loved ones. Their symptoms are severe enough to impact their daily activities.

Anxiety 2

1. B. Adjustment disorder

This patient presents with adjustment disorder with depressed mood after being informed of bad news. His symptoms have occurred within three months of the stressor.

2. C. Agoraphobia

This is a condition in which patients avoid places or people that might cause their symptoms of anxiety to become exacerbated.

3. J. Panic attack

These are brief episodes of intense anxiety in which patients may experience physical symptoms such as palpitations, shortness of breath and dizziness.

4. I. Obsessive compulsive disorder

This is an anxiety related condition which involves obsessions, compulsions or both. This condition can significantly impair an affected individual's daily activities

5. D. Body dysmorphic disorder

This is a condition in which an individual is obsessed about their body or appearance. The pre-occupation can lead to social anxiety and avoidance.

6. E. Dermatillomania

This is a condition which is characterised by a patient's urge to pick at their own skin, to the extent that it causes physical damage.

Behavioural conditions 1

1. B. Attention deficit hyperactivity disorder (ADHD)

Patients commonly present with high levels of activity, difficulty remaining still for prolonged periods of time and poor levels of attention. Their actions can impact their function at school, work and at home.

2. D. Borderline personality disorder

She has a pattern of unstable and intense interpersonal relationships, she has a persistently unstable self-image, inappropriate intense anger or rage, recurrent threats of self-harm and impulsivity in areas which are self-damaging (spending and driving in this case).

3. I. Oppositional defiant disorder

The correct answer is oppositional defiant disorder. This is a pattern of irritable mood, argumentative behaviour and vindictiveness which lasts for a period of at least six months.

4. A. Antisocial personality disorder

This patient has failure to conform to social norms, disregard for the rights of others and lack of remorse. He has evidence of conduct disorder with onset before 15.

Behavioural conditions 2

1. E. Conduct disorder

This patient is under the age of 18 and has demonstrated a repetitive and persistent pattern of behaviour in which the basic rights of others as well as societal norms or rules are violated.

2. G. Kleptomania

This is a condition in which individuals are unable to resist the urge to steal items they do not require. They gain pleasure from the theft and they have no underlying motives other than this for their actions.

3. C. Autism spectrum disorder

This is a complex condition which involves difficulties with communication, affected individuals usually follow particular routines and rituals which help them cope with stress. Deviations from regular routines can cause significant distress in the form of tantrums. Patients also usually have restricted interests in which they excel.

4. H. Malingering

This individual does not meet the criteria for Kleptomania as outlined in the DSM 5, he has made financial gains from his actions and has requested a medical certificate to help him avoid the legal consequences of his actions.

Memory 1

1. C. Frontotemporal dementia

This patient has behavioural changes and evidence of change in personality, they also have difficulty with visual recognition of items. Memory changes tend to happen much later.

2. H. Normal pressure hydrocephalus

This patient presents with the classic triad of symptoms associated with normal pressure hydrocephalus. She has cognitive impairment, difficulty walking and poor bladder control.

3. L. Vascular dementia

This patient has multiple risk factors including smoking, hypertension, hyperlipidaemia, type 2 diabetes mellitus and recent stroke. This patient is likely suffering from multi-infarct dementia with a step wise worsening of symptoms rather than a smooth progression of symptoms. This patient also exhibits asymmetric reflexes and pseudobulbar changes.

4. M. Wernicke's encephalopathy

This patient presents with acute mental status changes, nystagmus, evidence of liver failure and ataxia.

Memory 2

1. K. Neurosyphilis

This patient has presented with memory loss, personality changes and tabes dorsalis a late complication of syphilis. Tabes dorsalis includes locomotor

ataxia (tabetic gait), Argyll Robertson pupils, paraesthesia, bladder incontinence, diminished reflexes and tabetic ocular crises.

2. I. Parkinson's disease

This patient has typical features of Parkinson's disease including a shuffling
gait and cogwheel rigidity. Parkinson's disease not only affects motor function but can also affect the thought processes, memory and mental function
of the affected individual. This individual has features of Parkinson's disease
dementia.

3. E. Huntington's disease

This middle-aged patient has had a change in personality, involuntary jerking
movements and memory loss. Huntington's disease is a genetic condition which is
inherited in an autosomal dominant manner and the children of affected individuals have a 50% chance of inheriting the gene mutation and developing the condition. This patient also has CT brain findings consistent with Huntington's disease.

4. G. Lewy body dementia

This is a progressive dementia in which the affected individuals have decline in
mental function and often experience visual hallucinations.

Paraphilic conditions 1

1. F. Sexual masochism disorder

This patient has recurrent and intense sexual arousal from being humiliated and
beaten by sexual partners. This patient also engages in asphyxiophilia where
they derive sexual pleasure from restriction of breathing.

2. B. Fetishistic disorder

This patient derives intense sexual arousal from non-genital body parts and
non-living objects, in this case feet and shoes. He is unable to function in his
day-to-day life as a result of his feelings.

3. D. Paedophilic disorder – exclusive type

This individual has intense sexual fantasies involving a child below the age of
13 for at least six months, which are now causing him significant distress. He is
aged 16 and at least five years older than the individual.

4. I. Transvestic disorder with fetishism.

This person fantasises about cross dressing, derives intense sexual arousal from
these thoughts. He is very much aroused by feminine clothing and fabrics. His
thoughts and behaviours are impacting his work and social life.

Paraphilic conditions 2

1. C. Frotteuristic disorder

He has intense sexual arousal from touching or rubbing up against non-consenting individuals.

2. J. Voyeuristic disorder

He has had recurrent episodes of sexual arousal as a result of observing a non-
consenting individual while naked. The individual being observed is at least 18
at the time of the event.

3. G. Sexual sadism disorder

This patient achieves sexual pleasure from the suffering of others whether that be physical or psychological. This patient has also perpetrated these acts against a non-consenting individual.

4. A. Exhibitionistic disorder

This individual has been exposing himself to prepubertal children and physically mature individuals. He has been doing this for greater than six months He reports that he gets intense sexual arousal as a result of exposing himself to these individuals.

Personality disorders 1

1. H. Paranoid personality disorder

This patient is distrustful and suspicious of the motives of others, interpreting them as being malevolent.

2. B. Avoidant personality disorder

This patient has hypersensitivity to negative evaluation, a feeling of inadequacy and social inhibition.

3. E. Histrionic personality disorder

This patient has attention seeking qualities and is excessively emotional.

4. J. Schizotypal personality disorder

This patient has delusions of reference, eccentric behaviour, odd beliefs, paranoid ideations and discomfort in close relationships.

Personality disorders 2

1. D. Dependent personality disorder

This patient struggles to make every day decisions for herself, needs others to assume responsibility for her, feels helpless when alone and has sought another relationship as a source of care and support after her divorce.

2. A. Antisocial personality disorder

This patient has failure to conform to social norms, disregard for the rights of others and lack of remorse. He has evidence of conduct disorder with onset before 15.

3. I. Schizoid personality disorder

Patients usually have a restricted range of emotional expression and a pattern of detachment from social relationships.

4. F. Narcissistic personality disorder

This patient lacks empathy, seeks admiration from others and holds grandiose beliefs about themselves.

Substance related and Addictive disorders 1

1. K. Cocaine intoxication

This patient presents with agitation and anxiety. She also has physical signs of cocaine intoxication including tachycardia, hypertension, diaphoresis, nasal septum perforations and dilated pupils. An acute myocardial infarction can occur with cocaine intoxication, this case demonstrates an example of an inferior MI.

2. A. Alcohol intoxication
These individual expresses clinically problematic behaviour as evidenced by his aggressive behaviour. He also demonstrates slurred speech, unsteady gait and poor co-ordination with his driving.

3. H. Cannabis intoxication
This patient presents with classical features of cannabis intoxication including perceptual disturbances, tachycardia, dry mouth, increased appetite and conjunctival injection.

4. P. Phencyclidine (PCP) intoxication
This patient is agitated and assaulting others, he also demonstrates signs of intoxication such as tachycardia, hypertension, ataxia, muscle rigidity and horizontal nystagmus. Other signs or symptoms can include vertical nystagmus, numbness or diminishes pain response, dysarthria, seizure like activity and hyperacusis.

5. C. Alcohol withdrawal
This patient has evidence of autonomic hyperactivity (tachycardia and sweating), insomnia and anxiety.

Substance related and Addictive disorders 2

1. O. Opioid withdrawal
She is restless, anxious, has been suffering from gastrointestinal disturbances and has pupillary dilatation. Examination reveals rhinorrhoea and normal blood pressure with a raised heart rate.

2. M. Opioid intoxication
This patient is in a stupor, exhibits respiratory depression and present with pupillary constriction. Blood pressure can be reduced and pulmonary oedema can sometimes occur as demonstrated in this case.

3. F. Caffeine intoxication
He is restless, nervous and suffering from muscle twitching. His examination findings reveal psychomotor agitation, facial flushing and tachycardia which proceeds to an arrhythmia. It is likely that he has consumed an excessive amount of caffeine powder which has been added to his protein shake. Ventricular fibrillation is a common cause of death in caffeine overdose.

4. D. Amphetamine intoxication
This patient presents as a very energetic and talkative person with a decreased appetite. She also has tachycardia, hypertension, low grade fever, tachypnoea and dilated pupils.

Eating disorders 1

1. B. Avoidant restrictive food intake disorder
She has an eating disturbance as she is concerned about the adverse consequences of doing so. As a result of her food avoidance, she has had a significant loss of weight.

2. H. Pica
This patient has been eating non-food substances for over one month which is not a part of a socially normative practice.

3. F. Night eating syndrome

This patient has been having recurrent episodes of night eating which is causing him distress and affecting his daily function.

4. C. Binge eating disorder

She has recurrent episodes of binge eating in which she eats excessive amounts of food quickly and feels out of control with her eating habits. She is distressed by her symptoms and has no obvious inappropriate compensatory behaviour as seen in bulimia nervosa. She has episodes on average at least one day a week for more than a year.

Eating disorders 2

1. E. Kleine–Levin syndrome

This is a rare condition which can be associated with excessive periods of sleep, mood or behaviour changes, hyperphagia and abnormally increased sexual desire.

2. D. Bulimia nervosa

She has recurrent episodes of binge eating and feels as though she lacks control over her eating habits. She has inappropriate compensatory behaviours to prevent weight gain such as excessive exercise and potentially self-induced vomiting as evidenced by her enamel erosion. She has concerns about her body image and her episodes occur at least a couple of days a week for the past six months.

3. G. Orthorexia nervosa

This patient spends a great deal of time preparing his meals, feels he is more superior than others as a result of his diet and is very rigid with his dietary rules. His behaviours are affecting his relationships with those close to him.

4. A. Anorexia nervosa

She has restricted her dietary intake which has resulted in a significantly low body weight. She has a fear of weight gain despite her low weight and has disturbances in the way in which her body weight is experienced.

Neurology

4

CRANIAL NERVE PATHOLOGY

A. Abducent nerve
B. Accessory spinal nerve
C. Facial nerve
D. Glossopharyngeal nerve
E. Hypoglossal nerve
F. Oculomotor nerve
G. Olfactory nerve
H. Optic nerve
I. Trigeminal nerve
J. Trochlear nerve
K. Vagus nerve
L. Vestibulocochlear nerve

For each of the following, which nerve is MOST likely affected?

1. A 40-year-old plumber presents with a two-week history of shoulder and neck pain. He explains that his symptoms have become progressively worse and are now causing him difficulty sleeping. On examination he has an asymmetric neckline, atrophy of the trapezius on the right side, winging of the right scapula and weakness with forward elevation of the shoulder on the right.

2. A 31-year-old woman attends with a one-week history of left sided facial weakness. She explains that she has been finding it difficult to drink water during her workouts and is quite embarrassed by the fact that the water dribbles out of her mouth and down her face. Julie recently had a flu like illness a day before her symptoms started. On examination she has mild left sided facial droop.

3. A 59-year-old diabetic woman presents with a complaint of diplopia. She explains that her symptoms have been present for the past three days and are worse when she looks downward or when trying to read a book. On examination her right eye turns upward and outward when looking forward and elevates medially when looking left.

4. A 24-year-old presents three days after a high-speed car accident. He suffered from whiplash injury to his neck and facial injuries. He reports that he has had neck pain since the accident and over the past two days his sense of smell

has decreased. On examination his facial injuries have healed up well. You arrange for a CT scan of his brain and which reveals a small fracture affecting the ethmoid bone.

5. A 23-year-old university student presents complaining of numbness in her face for the past two days. On examination there is reduced sensation in the right forehead and the corneal reflex is absent on the same side.

6. A 16-year-old boy presents for review after tonsillectomy last week. He has not had any bleeding but explains that he has been suffering from dysgeusia affecting the posterior third of his tongue on the right side.

See page 101 for answers.

DIZZINESS

A. Acoustic neuroma
B. Benign paroxysmal positional vertigo (BPPV)
C. Labyrinthitis
D. Meniere's disease
E. Panic attack
F. Ramsay Hunt syndrome
G. Stroke
H. Vestibular migraine
I. Vestibular neuritis

For each of the following, what is the MOST likely diagnosis?

1. A 28-year-old woman was at work earlier today when she suddenly felt dizzy, noticed her heart begin to race, she felt tightness in her chest and reports that she felt short of breath. She presents at your emergency department where you review her. She has no significant medical history. You find no abnormality on physical examination.

2. A 37-year-old man presents with a complaint of dizziness. He reports that he has had a few episodes of dizziness over the past week associated with headaches. He has a long history of migraine like headaches which he treats with simple analgesia to good effect but has never had associated dizziness. He denies hearing loss or tinnitus and there are no significant examination findings.

3. A 26-year-old lady presents with a complaint of gradual onset of imbalance which has persisted for the past three days. Associated with this she has horizontal nystagmus at rest and left sided unilateral gradual hearing loss and tinnitus. One-week prior Louisa reports that she was treated with amoxicillin for acute otitis media associated with a fever.

4. A 72-year-old man presents with a one-day history of nausea and dizziness. He describes a sensation of "the room spinning around" which was constant and had left him bed bound last night. You review his patient notes and see that he had attended your clinic ten days prior for the management of herpes zoster affecting the right side of his chest, these symptoms have since settled. On examination he has fast beating horizontal nystagmus towards the right, the remainder of the neurological examination was unremarkable. He denies hearing loss.

5. A 78-year-old widow presents complaining of dizziness. She reports that over the past five days she has had an intermittent spinning sensation and has been feeling very nauseated. She reports that she had collapsed to the ground on one occasion but did not sustain any injuries, she is fearful that she may injure herself at home. She explains that the sensation is worse when turning over in the morning while in bed and when she bends over to pick things up. There is no associated tinnitus and she examines well.

See page 101 for answers.

EPILEPSY 1

A. **Absence seizure**
B. **Complex partial seizure**
C. **Dacrystic seizure**
D. **Dravet syndrome**
E. **Febrile seizure**
F. **Gelastic seizure**
G. **Hypnic myoclonus**
H. **Juvenile myoclonic epilepsy**
I. **Meningitis**
J. **Neonatal seizure**
K. **Pre-Eclampsia**
L. **Psychogenic non-epileptic seizures (PNES)**
M. **Simple partial seizure**
N. **Tonic-Clonic seizure**
O. **Tonic reflex seizures of early infancy**
P. **West syndrome**

For each of the following, what is the MOST likely diagnosis?

1. A 2-year-old girl is brought in by ambulance with her worried parents. The parents explain that 30 minutes ago she had collapsed to the ground at home and began to shake uncontrollably, the episode lasted three minutes and she was very

tired after this. She has been unwell for the past two days with a cough and runny nose, she had a temperature of 38.6°C last night which settled with Panadol.

2. A 4-year-old girl presents with her mother who is concerned about episodes of blanking out that she has been experiencing over the past month. She has episodes where she has become unresponsive while watching television or playing, during the episodes her eyes remain wide open, she returns to her activity after a few seconds and continues on as if she is unaware of what has happened.

3. A 21-year-old student attends with a complaint of ongoing right sided headache for the past two months. He is due for his final year examinations next week and believes his headache may be due to a combination of poor sleep and stress as he has been spending many hours awake studying. He is most concerned about jerky motions in his arms that he has been having in the past few days which are associated with the headaches. You refer him to a neurologist who performs a partial sleep deprivation EEG which reveals 3–6 Hz generalised poly-spike and wave discharges associated with myoclonic jerks early in the morning.

4. A 26-year-old student attends your clinic complaining of intermittent episodes of involuntary right lower limb movements over the past three months, on occasion he reports experiencing a burnt rubber smell associated with this. He has no history of similar and explains that he has had increasing episodes in the lead up to his final year assessments which are causing him much anxiety. He denies alteration of conscious state and has a full recollection of events.

5. A 24-year-old woman attends your emergency department via ambulance suffering from full body rigors. She was at her local GP clinic an hour ago for an influenza vaccination and shortly after the dose she developed full body shakes which came every five to ten minutes and each episode lasted for about a minute. She remained awake and conversant during episodes. On examination you find no evidence of injury and neurological examination is unremarkable. She has several episodes in the emergency department and is subsequently admitted to the neurology ward for observation. On the ward a video EEG demonstrates no significant changes prior to, during or after episodes.

6. A 6-month-old infant is brought in by her concerned parents. Over the past two days she has been having episodes of sudden flexion of her body, arms and legs. Episodes last for about two seconds then settle for about five seconds before occurring again. She has about ten to 15 episodes within each cluster and they occur two times a day. An EEG reveals typical features of hypsarrhythmia – high amplitude, asynchronous and arrhythmia.

See page 102 for answers.

EPILEPSY 2

A. **Absence seizure**
B. **Complex partial seizure**

C. Dacrystic seizure
D. Dravet syndrome
E. Febrile seizure
F. Gelastic seizure
G. Hypnic myoclonus
H. Juvenile myoclonic epilepsy
 I. Meningitis
J. Neonatal seizure
K. Pre-Eclampsia
L. Psychogenic non-epileptic seizures (PNES)
M. Simple partial seizure
N. Tonic-Clonic seizure
O. Tonic reflex seizures of early infancy
P. West syndrome

For each of the following, what is the MOST likely diagnosis?

1. A 32-year-old male was found by a colleague seated in his car outside of his workplace. His colleague was concerned as she reports James was behaving quite strangely, flapping his arms and hitting his steering wheel quite violently. She knocked on his window but he did not respond to her. An ambulance was called and on arrival 15 minutes later he had become responsive but was quite lethargic. He cannot recall how he had arrived in the car park, the last thing he remembers was "the smell of burning rubber" after having gotten into his car at home.

2. A 26-year-old pregnant woman, G1P0, presents with a two-day history of headache, she explains that it is generalised and mildly uncomfortable. Jodie is currently 26 weeks' gestation. She took her blood pressure last night at home on her father's blood pressure device and had a reading of 164/92 mmHg, she thought the elevation may have been due to anxiety and the pain of the headache. Jodie decided to sleep on it and see you in the morning. You take her blood pressure today which reads 167/93 mmHg. Her last reading two weeks ago was 120/84. You perform a urine dipstick which reveals proteinuria 2+.

3. A 34-year-old man presents to your clinic with his partner who explains that she is concerned about him as he has been having sudden jerking motions of his arms and legs in his bed at night. His symptoms occur shortly after he falls asleep and have been waking his partner up at night.

4. A 15-day-old child is brought into the emergency department by her worried mother who explains that she became very stiff in all of her limbs for about two minutes and had associated jerking motions. Mum noticed her having small jerking motions while being breastfed since she was born, but not as bad as they were today. The pregnancy was uneventful and she was born at term without complication, she is only breastfed and has had no recent illness. On examination she has a temperature of 36.8°C, weighs 3.1 kg and is in the 50th centile for head circumference and length. Examination is otherwise unremarkable.

5. A 64-year-old man is brought into your emergency department by ambulance after suffering from a medical episode at home. His daughter tells you that he was helping her hang a mirror, she left the room to collect a tool when she heard a loud noise and the sound of glass breaking. Rachel immediately returned to the room where she found him unresponsive and writhing about on the floor, she safely removed the shattered mirror from around him and called an ambulance. The episode lasted for ten minutes and she reports that he was very fatigued after this. Examination is unremarkable.

See pages 102–103 for answers.

FACIAL PAIN

A. **Acute rhinosinusitis**
B. **Chronic rhinosinusitis with polyps**
C. **Chronic rhinosinusitis without polyps**
D. **Eagle's syndrome**
E. **Glossopharyngeal neuralgia**
F. **Greater occipital neuralgia**
G. **Post-Herpetic trigeminal neuropathy**
H. **Sialolithiasis**
I. **Temporal arteritis**
J. **Temporomandibular joint dysfunction**
K. **Trigeminal neuralgia**

For each of the following, what is the MOST likely diagnosis?

1. A 47-year-old male attends with a two-year history of intermittent left sided sharp lancinating facial pain affecting his jaw and cheek. He reports that the episodes last for about 30 seconds and then settle. He reports that episodes are usually triggered by eating. Examination is unremarkable and he is asymptomatic on review.
2. A 31-year-old woman presents with left sided facial pain and swelling. She explains that her symptoms are worse just before meals and when eating food. On examination you can palpate a lump in the buccal mucosa on the left side of the mouth.
3. A 21-year-old male presents with a six-day history of thick green nasal discharge, left sided facial pain and a fever. He explains that his symptoms initially started with a sore throat and dry cough which resolved after two days, he improved slightly but his situation then began to deteriorate. On examination he has a temperature of 38.6°C, facial pain on percussion over the left cheek and pressure in the same location on leaning forward.
4. A 70-year-old man presents with left sided headache and jaw pain associated with visual impairment. He explains that his pain has been there for the past

two weeks and is worse with meals. On examination he is tender on palpation of the left side of his head.

5. A 24-year-old science student attends with right sided jaw pain, he reports that he has had this pain for the past two years. He tells you that the pain is occasionally associated with a loud popping sound on the right side when opening his mouth. On examination there is crepitus palpable anterior to the right ear with depression of the mandible.

6. A 55-year-old pianist attends with a three-year history of intermittent stabbing pain on the left occipital area of his head and occasional radiation to the fronto-orbital area on the left. He reports that the symptoms last for most of the day and were worse during the night. He reports that when he wears tight fitting caps his symptoms are usually evoked.

See page 103 for answers.

HEADACHE 1

A. **Acephalgic migraine**
B. **Arnold–Chiari malformation**
C. **Brain abscess**
D. **Cluster headache**
E. **Ice pick headache**
F. **Idiopathic intracranial hypertension**
G. **Low CSF headache**
H. **Medication overuse headache**
I. **Medulloblastoma**
J. **Meningitis**
K. **Migraine**
L. **Migraine with aura**
M. **Reversible cerebral vasoconstriction syndrome**
N. **Status migrainosus**
O. **Subarachnoid haemorrhage**
P. **Tension headache**

For each of the following, what is the MOST likely diagnosis?

1. A 53-year-old presents with a five-month history of sudden, intensely sharp and painful stabbing sensations across the top of his head. The sensations last for a few seconds and have no particular pattern. On some days he will have ten to 20 similar episodes and on others he will have none, he has no associated symptoms. Neurological examination is unremarkable so too are investigations including an MRI brain.

2. A 34-year-old woman reports a six-month history of headaches, she explains that episodes occur at least three or four times a week and she feels a band like

pressure radiating around her whole head. Episodes last for about one hour before settling with simple analgesia.

3. A 42-year-old man presents with a three-day history of headache. He reports that his headache is very severe when he is sitting upright or standing, is mostly at the back of his head and associated with neck pain. He explains that his symptoms resolve quickly when he lays down flat. He has a history of thoracic spinal stenosis and has had a laminectomy for treatment of this five days ago.

4. A 31-year-old nurse attends complaining of deep sharp pain around her right eye, it is associated with drooping of the right upper eyelid, tearing and a running nose. She explains that she has had five episodes since this morning and was awoken by the initial episode.

5. A 22-year-old woman presents with a two-week history of headache associated with binocular diplopia. On examination she has a BMI of 37 and fundoscopy reveals papilledema.

See page 103 for answers.

HEADACHE 2

A. **Acephalgic migraine**
B. **Arnold–Chiari malformation**
C. **Brain abscess**
D. **Cluster headache**
E. **Ice pick headache**
F. **Idiopathic intracranial hypertension**
G. **Low CSF headache**
H. **Medication overuse headache**
 I. **Medulloblastoma**
 J. **Meningitis**
K. **Migraine**
L. **Migraine with aura**
M. **Reversible cerebral vasoconstriction syndrome**
N. **Status migrainosus**
O. **Subarachnoid haemorrhage**
P. **Tension headache**

For each of the following, what is the MOST likely diagnosis?

1. A 29-year-old accountant attends with pain on the right side of her head for the past six hours. The pain is sharp, pulsating in nature and is associated with photophobia. She has a long history of similar such headaches and reports that she has been having an increased frequency of these over the past four months.

She denies visual disturbances, has not had any recent illness, she has a history of acne for which she is on the oral contraceptive pill and takes no other regular medication. Examination is unremarkable. She requests a script for Rizatriptan, she has been using these on a daily basis over this period of time and has found relief with them.

2. A 54-year-old migraineur attends with sudden onset severe headache. It is the worst headache he has ever had and not similar to his regular migraine headaches. On examination he has neck stiffness and is unable to extend his knee when his hip and knee are flexed to 90 degrees and he is supine. You arrange for an urgent CT scan of the brain.

3. A 12-year-old boy attends with a headache for the past two hours which is associated with a fever, he is covering his eyes as he cannot look into the light. On examination he has a temperature of 38.9°C, there is a widespread non blanching maculopapular rash across his body and Kernig's sign is positive.

4. A 37-year-old male has been in bed for the past four days with a left sided headache, he has had no fevers, no recent illness or recent travel. He reports that he has had similar such headaches in the past and has been given IM Morphine with good results. NSAIDs and paracetamol have been ineffective during the current episode. On examination he has a temperature of 36.5°C, no neck stiffness and no rash. Cranial nerves and neurological examination were unremarkable.

5. A 19-year-old university student presents with a left sided headache for the past eight hours which was preceded by zigzag shaped bright lights in the lower visual field of her left eye, she explains that it is similar to previous headaches she has had and usually settles with rest. She has no significant medical history and takes no regular medication. Neurological examination is unremarkable.

See page 104 for answers.

HEARING LOSS 1

A. **Acute otitis media**
B. **Barotrauma**
C. **Cerumen impaction**
D. **Cholesteatoma**
E. **Eustachian tube dysfunction**
F. **Exostosis**
G. **Glomus tumor**
H. **Otosclerosis**
I. **Otitis externa**
J. **Ototoxicity**
K. **Vestibular schwannoma**

For each of the following, what is the MOST likely diagnosis?

1. A 23-year-old woman presents with pain in her left ear and reduced hearing. She explains that her symptoms started the day prior to attendance and have progressively worsened overnight, she has also had a runny nose and has had rigors. On examination she has a temperature of 38.1°C and she has a bulging left tympanic membrane.

2. A 43-year-old man presents with bilateral hearing impairment. He reports that hearing loss was first noted in the left ear two days ago but is now also affecting the right ear. He has a history of hypertension and erectile dysfunction; he is on Perindopril and has been using Sildenafil daily for the past two weeks. On otoscopic examination you find no abnormality.

3. A 12-year-old has a three-year history of progressive hearing loss in his right ear. He reports that he has also been suffering from tinnitus during this period of time. Otoscopic examination reveals a positive Schwartz sign in the right ear.

4. A 39-year-old presents with reduced hearing in her left ear for the past four days. On otoscopic examination you note left sided hemotypanum and a normal external ear exam. She flew home from a conference she was attending in India and her symptoms started shortly after this.

5. A 45-year-old man presents with a three-month history of foul-smelling purulent discharge from his right ear, this associated with decreased hearing and a feeling of fullness within the affected ear. He has not experienced any pain or vertigo. On otoscopic examination you note a brown coloured irregular mass within the external auditory canal.

See page 104 for answers.

HEARING LOSS 2

A. Acute otitis media
B. Barotrauma
C. Cerumen impaction
D. Cholesteatoma
E. Eustachian tube dysfunction
F. Exostosis
G. Glomus tumor
H. Otosclerosis
 I. Otitis externa
J. Ototoxicity
K. Vestibular schwannoma

For each of the following, what is the MOST likely diagnosis?

1. A 36-year-old man presents with a three-day history of muffled hearing in his left ear associated with pressure and a feeling of fullness. There is no history of trauma and he has not experienced any discharge from the ear. He has a history of recurrent ear infections and hay fever. He is afebrile and otoscopic examination is normal. You organise for tympanometry which reveals he has a type C tympanogram.

2. A 6-year-old girl attends your clinic with her mother. She tells you that she has a painful left ear, which is very itchy and associated with reduced hearing. Her symptoms started three days ago after she went swimming with her siblings. She is tender with movement of the tragus and pinna, otoscopic exam reveals a swollen and closed external auditory canal. Weber's test lateralises to the left side and Rinne's test reveals bone conduction being better than air conduction.

3. A 43-year-old surfer presents complaining of reduced hearing in bilateral ears. He explains that it has been worsening over the past six months. He tells you that over the past few years he has struggled to remove water from his ears when goes surfing. On examination he has several skin covered masses within the canals bilaterally.

4. A 67-year-old woman presents to with a five-month history of progressively worsening hearing loss in her right ear. She complains of a ringing sensation in the affected ear during this time. Over the past two days she has become very dizzy, this has worried her greatly as the episodes lasted for several hours. Physical examination reveals sensorineural hearing loss affecting the right ear, right sided facial droop and absent corneal reflex on the same side.

5. A 45-year-old lecturer presents with a two-day history of hearing loss. You arrange for tympanometry which reveals a type B tympanogram with low volume.

See page 105 for answers.

MOVEMENT DISORDERS 1

A. Acute dystonia
B. Akathisia
D. Essential tremor
E. Huntington's disease
F. Neuroleptic malignant syndrome
G. Parkinsonism
H. Parkinson's disease
I. Serotonin syndrome
J. Sydenham chorea
K. Tardive dyskinesia
L. Tourette's syndrome

For each of the following, what is the MOST likely diagnosis?

1. A 46-year-old schizophrenic male patient is admitted to the psychiatric ward at your local rural hospital, he was initially commenced on Haloperidol 5 mg IM two times a day for treatment of auditory and visual hallucinations. The chart was recently re-written two days ago by a locum doctor and you note that there is an increase in the dose of the Haloperidol now making it QID without any clear written progress notes to document why the change has occurred. The nurse in charge of the ward is concerned that there may have been a medication error and has called you to assess him as he now has muscle stiffness. On review the patient is non-verbal, has lead pipe rigidity in both upper and lower limbs and marked diaphoresis. He has a temperature 38.9°C, HR 122, BP 132/84 mmHg and RR 20. Laboratory investigations reveal CK 1556, WCC 19, kidney and liver function tests are within normal limits.

2. A 47-year-old presents with a long history of shakes in his hands. His symptoms are worse when his hands are outstretched but absent when he is at rest, his father had similar symptoms. He explains that he occasionally has a glass of wine at work to help with his symptoms. On examination he has a symmetrical hand tremor which is not present at rest, examination is otherwise unremarkable.

3. A 38-year-old presents with a migraine headache, he was commenced on IV Chlorpromazine in the emergency department. Shortly after the commencement of the medication he began to complain of a tremor in his hands which rapidly progressed to rigidity and bradykinesia.

4. A 39-year-old presents with a six-month history of writhing and jerking movements in her limbs which are making her routines more difficult to perform. Her mother explains that her personality has changed in recent months and that she has become easily agitated. Her father had similar symptoms and passed away at the age of 48. On examination you note involuntary irregular movements of the upper limbs.

See page 105 for answers.

MOVEMENT DISORDERS 2

A. **Acute dystonia**
B. **Akathisia**
C. **Creutzfeldt–Jakob disease**
D. **Essential tremor**
E. **Huntington's disease**
F. **Neuroleptic malignant syndrome**
G. **Parkinsonism**
H. **Parkinson's disease**

I. Serotonin syndrome
J. Sydenham chorea
K. Tardive dyskinesia
L. Tourette's syndrome

For each of the following, what is the MOST likely diagnosis?

1. A 32-year-old presents with a three-day history of worsening body aches, palpitations, severe fatigue, uncontrollable twitching and tremors. She has a history of depression and has been on fluoxetine 20 mg daily for a year without issue. She reports that she commenced St John's wort six months ago by her naturopath. Four days ago, she had a migraine while at a friend's house and used some of her Tramadol to manage it, she continued this for the next day and stopped after her symptoms began.

2. An 82-year-old resident of the local residential aged care facility is brought into your emergency department. He has been suffering from dysphagia and abnormal tongue protrusions which had progressively worsened over the past two hours. You review his medication chart and note that he was commenced on Haloperidol by a locum doctor as he had been restless for the past few days. On examination he has bite marks on his tongue and stiffness in the masseter muscles.

3. A 72-year-old woman reports that she has become unsteady on her feet and has had four falls at home in the past 12 months. Fortunately, she has not suffered significant injury as a result of these falls. As she enters your room you note that she walks in a shuffling motion. On examination she has marked cogwheel rigidity and bradykinesia in her upper limbs without obvious tremor, she also has brisk reflexes in her lower limbs.

4. A 32-year-old reports a long history of repetitive involuntary movements, since childhood, that are exacerbated by stressful situations. He explains that he was recently promoted at work and has taken on additional responsibilities including weekly team meetings in which he has to present in front of colleagues. He reports that during these presentations he has had an increased amount of jerking motions, blinking and sniffing movements. He feels increasingly embarrassed by these behaviours.

See pages 105–106 for answers.

NEUROMUSCULAR DISORDERS 1

A. Acute brachial neuritis
B. Acute inflammatory polyradiculoneuropathy
C. Bell's palsy

D. Charcot–Marie–Tooth disease
E. Duchenne muscular dystrophy
F. Inclusion body myositis
G. Kennedy's syndrome
H. Motor neurone disease
 I. Multiple sclerosis
 J. Myasthenia gravis
K. Parkinson's disease
L. Syringomyelia

For each of the following, what is the MOST likely diagnosis?

1. A 33-year-old librarian presents with muscle fatigue and clumsiness. She has been struggling to hold books at work and has also had difficulty with her gait, falling twice in the past six months. She has also had worsening vision over the past 12 months. On brain MRI you see Dawson's fingers. You arrange for visual evoked potential testing which demonstrates slowed conduction in optic nerves, a spinal tap reveals oligoclonal bands in the CSF.

2. A 38-year-old attends with right sided facial drooping. He explains that he had had a flu like illness five days ago and that his symptoms had finally settled the day before. Yesterday he noticed it was difficult to close his right eye, his symptoms have progressed to complete right sided facial droop over the course of the past 24 hours. Examination reveals a right sided facial droop, cranial nerve exam reveals weakness of the 7th cranial nerve, all other cranial nerves examined were fine. You arrange for a CT brain which reveals no abnormalities.

3. A 58-year-old male presents to your clinic after having had a fall at home. He has had two other falls in the past six months. On presentation he is able to ambulate, but you note that he does so with a shuffling motion. On examination he has pronounced bradykinesia in his upper limbs associated with cogwheel rigidity.

4. A 51-year-old complains of chronic weakness in both his upper limbs, particularly in his fingers, for at least the past six years. On examination of his limbs, you observe atrophy of the musculature in his forearms and between his fingers, sensation and reflexes are preserved. You arrange for further investigations which reveal CK of 2653 (45–250 U/L). Electromyography demonstrates complex repetitive discharges associated with fibrillation while at rest and low amplitude, short duration motor unit potentials with contraction. You arrange for a biopsy which confirms your diagnosis.

See page 106 for answers.

NEUROMUSCULAR DISORDERS 2

A. Acute brachial neuritis
B. Acute inflammatory polyradiculoneuropathy
C. Bell's palsy
D. Charcot–Marie–Tooth disease
E. Duchenne muscular dystrophy
F. Inclusion body myositis
G. Kennedy's syndrome
H. Motor neurone disease
 I. Multiple sclerosis
 J. Myasthenia gravis
K. Parkinson's disease
L. Syringomyelia

For each of the following, what is the MOST likely diagnosis?

1. A 46-year-old complains of a three-month history of weakness in her right arm and difficulty holding her tools while at work, frequently losing grip of them. She feels clumsy while walking at times but has had no falls, she also reports muscle twitching and cramps in her arms and legs. On examination you note atrophy of the musculature of the right arm when compared to the left, you also note fasciculations in both the upper and lower limbs. Power and reflexes are reduced in the right upper limb. Co-ordination is intact. Cranial nerve examination was unremarkable.

2. A 68-year-old presents with worsening dysphagia to both fluids and solids over the past two months. He reports that he has lost 5 kg in the past month, his partner has also noticed that he has had droopy eyelids since his symptoms first began. He has a past history of dyslipidaemia and hypertension. Examination reveals bilateral eyelid ptosis, reduced muscle strength in his upper limbs bilaterally and reflexes are preserved.

3. A 5-year-old boy presents as he has had multiple falls in the past three months. On examination he has a waddling gait, lumbar hyper-lordosis, he is walking on his toes and has marked calf hypertrophy. Gower's sign is positive.

4. A 14-year-old boy attends with his mother who is concerned about his posture and clumsiness. He feels weak in all of his limbs and especially his lower limbs. He has rolled his ankles several times this year as a result of his symptoms. On examination he walks with a high stepping gait and his feet slap the floor while he walks, you note muscle wasting in his lower limbs and high foot arches.

See page 106 for answers.

VISION LOSS 1

A. Acute angle closure glaucoma
B. Amaurosis fugax
C. Central retinal artery occlusion
D. Central retinal vein occlusion
E. Giant cell arteritis
F. Iritis
G. Keratitis
H. Macular degeneration
 I. Posterior vitreous detachment
 J. Primary open angle glaucoma
K. Retinal detachment
L. Retinitis pigmentosa

For each of the following, what is the MOST likely diagnosis?

1. A 15-year-old presents with visual loss. Over the past six months her vision has become very poor at night and she now struggles to get around her room when the lights are off. On fundus examination you note attenuated retinal arterioles, a pale optic disc and bone spicule pigmentation.

2. A 32-year-old presents with left eye pain. She wears contact lenses and forgot to remove them last night when she went to bed. She has had blurred vision and photophobia since this morning. On examination she has mucopurulent discharge from the left eye and fluorescein staining reveals multiple regions of brilliant green discoloration on the cornea.

3. A 63-year-old presents with his wife who is concerned that he has become clumsier. She explains that he has been bumping into objects about the house and has had two falls in the past six months. You send him to the local optometry clinic for an eye check. Tonometry is performed which reveals elevated IOP in both eyes with the right measuring 26 mmHg and the left measuring 32 mmHg. Fundoscopy examination reveals pale and cupped optic discs with retinal vessels displaced nasally on the surface of the disc. Visual field examination reveals peripheral vision loss.

4. A 72-year-old man presents with visual changes affecting his left eye. He explains that he can see black spots, like ants, moving about and affecting his vision. The symptoms are worsening and are associated with flashes of light. He has a history of hypertension, COPD and cataract surgery on his left eye.

5. A 51-year-old presents with a two-month history of worsening blurred vision in his right eye. On dilated fundoscopy examination you observe optic disc oedema and diffuse "blood and thunder" retinal haemorrhages.

6. An 80-year-old presents with sudden onset, painless, left sided vision loss. He explains that he saw a black spot in his vision which quickly covered his visual field in the left eye. He has a past history of hypertension, hyperlipidaemia and coronary artery disease. On fundoscopy examination you note a cherry red spot.

See page 107 for answers.

VISION LOSS 2

A. **Acute angle closure glaucoma**
B. **Amaurosis fugax**
C. **Central retinal artery occlusion**
D. **Central retinal vein occlusion**
E. **Giant cell arteritis**
F. **Iritis**
G. **Keratitis**
H. **Macular degeneration**
I. **Posterior vitreous detachment**
J. **Primary open angle glaucoma**
K. **Retinal detachment**
L. **Retinitis pigmentosa**

For each of the following, what is the MOST likely diagnosis?

1. A 68-year-old presents with left eye pain and blurred vision. She explains that she can see bright lights and rainbow-coloured halos in her left eye. The pain, which started three hours ago, is severe and radiating to her forehead. On examination she has an erythematous left eye with a dilated pupil which does not respond to light. Intraocular pressure (IOP) in the left eye is 52 mmHg.
2. A 24-year-old presents with a one-day history of pain in his left eye which has gradually worsened. The pain is associated with blurred vision and photophobia. He has a six-year history of lower back pain and uses simple analgesia for treatment of this. On examination he has an irregular miotic pupil and limbal flush affecting the left eye.
3. A 67-year-old presents complaining of a five-day history of right sided headache which is associated with decreased vision on the affected side which started yesterday. On examination he is tender on palpation of the right side of his head.
4. A 70-year-old woman presents complaining of changes in her vision. She noticed a black spot in the centre of her right visual field three weeks ago. She has a history of T2DM, hypertension and hyperlipidaemia. On fundoscopy examination you note scattered soft drusen. Amsler grid test reveals a blurred spot near the centre of the grid with wavy lines.

5. A 54-year-old man presents with sudden loss of vision in his right eye for the past 30 minutes. He explains that his vision disappeared just like a "black curtain coming down vertically". Shortly after arrival his vision returns. On examination his temperature is 36.1°C, BP 122/84 mmHg, respiratory rate 16 breaths per minute and heart rate of 78 beats per minute. Fundoscopy reveals no abnormality.

6. A 70-year-old presents with a two-day history of flashing lights and floaters in her left eye. On slit lamp examination you note "tobacco dust" in anterior vitreous.

See page 107 for answers.

ANSWERS

Cranial nerve pathology

1. B. Accessory spinal nerve
Common features are neckline asymmetry, trapezius muscle atrophy, winging of the scapula and muscle weakness on the affected side.

2. C. Facial nerve
Also known as Bell's palsy, this condition involves paralysis of the muscles on one side of the face. In most cases there is no identifiable aetiology, infection is believed to be a common cause.

3. J. Trochlear nerve
This patient has presented with vertical diplopia and typical exam findings of right sided trochlear nerve palsy.

4. G. Olfactory nerve
Olfactory loss after a head injury is a common occurrence as a result of injury to the brain. The olfactory nerve passes through small foramina in the cribriform plate which is part of the ethmoid bone. Fractures to the ethmoid bone can cause anosmia.

5. I. Trigeminal nerve
This patient has reduced sensation in the forehead as a result of involvement of ophthalmic division of the trigeminal nerve. The corneal reflex is also absent and this involves sensation of stimulus via the nasociliary branch of the ophthalmic division of the trigeminal nerve.

6. D. Glossopharyngeal nerve
The lingual branch of the glossopharyngeal nerve is at risk of injury during tonsillectomy and can result in dysgeusia in the posterior third of the tongue on the affected side if injury occurs.

Dizziness

1. E. Panic attack
This patient has presented with features consistent with a panic attack including; dizziness, tachycardia, chest tightness and shortness of breath. There are no obvious physical features consistent with any of the other listed diagnoses.

2. H. Vestibular migraine
Vestibular migraine can cause vertigo, visual disturbances and hearing changes. It is not always associated with a headache. It is the second most common cause of vertigo.

3. C. Labyrinthitis
Labyrinthitis is a common complication of otitis media, symptoms can include nausea, dizziness and hearing loss.

4. I. Vestibular neuritis
Patients with this condition typically present with a history of acute onset nausea and vertigo. Hearing remains intact. The condition usually resolves spontaneously.

5. B. Benign paroxysmal positional vertigo (BPPV)

You should suspect this diagnosis when vertigo is triggered by head movements. The diagnosis is confirmed when the Hallpike manoeuvre triggers the same symptoms.

Epilepsy 1

1. E. Febrile seizure

Febrile seizures generally occur in children aged between 3 months and 6 years. Seizures usually spontaneously resolve within 3 minutes.

2. A. Absence seizure

This is a form of epilepsy in which the individual blanks out and stares into space, these episodes last between 5 and 30 seconds followed by sudden return of awareness. These types of seizures are mostly seen in children.

3. H. Juvenile myoclonic epilepsy

This is the most common form of idiopathic generalised epilepsy in adults despite its misleading name. Myoclonic seizures are instant and short-lived contractions of muscles which can occur as a single contraction, repeated contractions or they can be continuous contractions. JME diagnosis is aided with an EEG, it reveals a very specific pattern known as a 3–6 Hz generalised poly-spike and wave discharge.

4. M. Simple partial seizure

This patient has presented with a history of simple partial seizure. With this type of seizure patients typically retain awareness, unlike complex partial seizures where there is an absence of awareness. During these episodes patients may not be able to control their motor function but they recall the events very well.

5. L. Psychogenic non-epileptic seizures (PNES)

PNES are episodes which appear as epilepsy but do not involve any change in the brain's electrical activity. PNES can be caused by traumatic events. Video EEG is the best test for diagnosis of PNES.

6. P. West syndrome

This child presents with spasms and hypsarrhythmia on EEG, therefore the most likely diagnosis in this situation is West syndrome.

Epilepsy 2

1. B. Complex partial seizure

This patient has presented with a first episode of complex partial seizure (also known as a focal onset impaired awareness seizure). With this type of seizure patients typically have a sudden absence of awareness, they may not be able to control their motor function and may not recall the events during the episode.

2. K. Pre-Eclampsia

This patient is presenting with pre-eclampsia, she has a persistently elevated blood pressure, neurological symptoms (headache) and proteinuria. She requires prompt review and management for her presentation.

3. G. Hypnic myoclonus

Also known as sleep myoclonus, patients suffer from sudden twitching movements while asleep.

4. J. Neonatal seizure

Neonatal seizures occur within the first 28 days of life and are most commonly caused by intracranial haemorrhages, perinatal ischaemic strokes and hypoxic-ischaemic encephalopathy. The seizures must be stopped as quickly as possible.

5. N. Tonic-Clonic seizure

This patient presents with what is assumed to be a tonic-clonic seizure, the event was unwitnessed and as such it is not known whether the presentation was a focal or generalised onset seizure.

Facial pain

1. K. Trigeminal neuralgia

Patients typically present with sudden shock like pain radiating through the distribution of one of the three divisions of the trigeminal nerve. First line treatment involves the use of Carbamazepine.

2. H. Sialolithiasis

This results from calcified masses which form within the salivary glands. Patients complain of facial pain and swelling especially when there is excessive saliva production, commonly when eating or prior to commencement of meals as a result of aromas that stimulate saliva production.

3. A. Acute rhinosinusitis

The acute form of rhinosinusitis lasts less than 4 weeks, chronic is defined as greater than 12 weeks.

4. I. Temporal arteritis

This condition affects the external carotid artery and associated branches, patients typically describe headache and jaw pain on the affected side. Visual loss can occur as a result of ischemia affecting the optic nerve.

5. J. Temporomandibular joint dysfunction

This can result from inflammation, degenerative processes, trauma or overuse. Patients present with a wide range of symptoms including jaw pain, ear pain and pain on mastication.

6. F. Greater occipital neuralgia

In this condition irritation of the greater occipital nerve anywhere along its distribution can cause sharp, sudden, tingling sensations typically on one side of the head.

Headache 1

1. E. Ice pick headache

Such headaches are painful, sudden and very severe, they are commonly described as stabbing like pain.

2. P. Tension headache

These are a common form of headache and are typically described as being band like in nature.

3. G. Low CSF headache

This type of headache is caused by CSF leakage, in this case the likely aetiology is recent spinal surgery.

4. D. Cluster headache

This type of headache occurs in clusters and is considerably painful for the affected individual. It can awaken a patient from their sleep at night, is usually focused around one eye and the head on the affected side.

5. F. Idiopathic intracranial hypertension

This is a common cause of papilledema in obese women of child bearing age.

Headache 2

1. H. Medication overuse headache

This patient has been using a triptan for greater than ten days per month. Patients taking opioids or triptans for more than ten days per month are at risk of medication overuse headaches. Nonopioid analgesia (paracetamol, NSAIDs) if used for more than 15 days per month can also cause these headaches.

2. O. Subarachnoid haemorrhage

This is a well-recognised cause for a "thunderclap" headache. This headache is considered a medical emergency and results from bleeding within the subarachnoid space which is normally filled with CSF.

3. J. Meningitis

This is a life-threatening condition which involves inflammation of the meninges that cover the brain and the spinal cord. This patient has typical examination features including a positive Kernig's sign which is pathognomonic for meningitis.

4. N. Status migrainosus

This is an example of status migrainosus where the migraine headache has lasted for greater than 72 hours.

5. L. Migraine with aura

This is a migraine associated with sensory disturbances including visual changes or sensory changes in the body.

Hearing loss 1

1. A. Acute otitis media

This painful condition occurs when the area behind the ear drum, known as the middle ear, becomes infected.

2. J. Ototoxicity

This patient has hearing loss secondary to sildenafil use. Sildenafil is a medication commonly prescribed for erectile dysfunction. Other common ototoxic drugs include; aminoglycoside antibiotics, NSAIDs, loop diuretics and platinum-based chemotherapy agents.

3. H. Otosclerosis

Schwartz sign is indicative of otosclerosis as the likely diagnosis, this is pink discoloration of the promontory which is as a result of increased vascularity. Schwartz sign is also known as the flamingo pink blush.

4. B. Barotrauma

Otic barotrauma is pain in the ear or tympanic membrane damage as a result of exposure to sudden pressure changes such. This is commonly experienced by those involved in diving or air travel.

5. D. Cholesteatoma

This is a benign skin lined cyst that arises from the middle ear, behind the ear drum. Those affected usually describe painless discharge from the affected ear, decreased hearing and vertigo.

Hearing loss 2

1. E. Eustachian tube dysfunction

The eustachian tube connects the pharynx to the middle ear. This eustachian tube helps to equalise pressure within the middle ear. When the eustachian tube is blocked hearing may become muffled and the ear may also feel full. Type C tympanogram is highly suggestive of eustachian tube dysfunction.

2. I. Otitis externa

This patient has clinical evidence of otitis externa and also has conductive hearing loss in their affected ear.

3. F. Exostosis

Also known as surfer's ear, these are benign growths of bone within the ear canals that result from repetitive exposure to cold water.

4. K. Vestibular schwannoma

Patients typically present with gradual unilateral hearing loss associated with tinnitus. If the schwannoma enlarges it can cause compression of the facial nerve resulting in facial nerve palsy and reduced or absent corneal reflex on the affected side.

5. C. Cerumen impaction

Cerumen within the auditory canal can impair hearing and should be removed before further investigation. A type B tympanogram with low volume is suggestive of this diagnosis.

Movement disorders 1

1. F. Neuroleptic malignant syndrome

The correct answer is neuroleptic malignant syndrome. This is a life-threatening condition that requires urgent treatment. It is caused by the use of antipsychotic agents such as Haloperidol.

2. D. Essential tremor

The correct answer is essential tremor. This is a neurological disorder which can cause involuntary shaking in the body. This occurs particularly in the hands and makes simple activities difficult for the affected individual.

3. G. Parkinsonism

The correct answer is Parkinsonism. Parkinsonism is any condition which causes movement disorders seen in Parkinson's disease such as: tremors, bradykinesia and muscle stiffness. This patient has presented with drug induced Parkinsonism caused by chlorpromazine, a first-generation antipsychotic.

6. E. Huntington's disease

This inherited neurodegenerative condition is associated with personality changes, characteristic jerking movements and a family history of similar.

Movement disorders 2

1. I. Serotonin syndrome
This is an emergency presentation and requires urgent treatment. It is caused by a build-up of serotonin in the body. This patient is using fluoxetine (an SSRI), St John's wort and tramadol (an opioid). The combination of these agents has caused this patient's presentation.

2. A. Acute dystonia
This patient has presented with acute dystonia after administration of a first-generation antipsychotic (Haloperidol).

3. H. Parkinson's disease
This is a progressive neuro-degenerative disorder which causes movement difficulties in affected individuals. It mostly affects dopamine producing neurons in the substantia nigra, a basal ganglia structure in the mid-brain.

4. L. Tourette syndrome
The patient has Tourette syndrome and has tics as part of this, the most appropriate first line management for his symptoms is clonidine.

Neuromuscular disorders 1

1. I. Multiple sclerosis
MS is an autoimmune condition which results in damage to the central nervous system (CNS). This patient has typical MRI findings. Visual evoked potential testing measures how long it takes for a visual stimulus to reach the occipital cortex and this can be delayed as a result of MS. Oligoclonal banding on CSF exam suggests inflammation in the CNS and is indicative of MS.

2. C. Bell's palsy
In this condition there is paralysis of the muscles on one side of the face. In most cases there is no identifiable aetiology, infection is believed to be a common cause.

3. K. Parkinson's disease
This is a progressive neurological condition that occurs as a result of reduced dopamine levels in the brain. Patients with this condition present with movement disorders including bradykinesia, muscle rigidity, tremor and shuffling gait.

4. F. Inclusion body myositis
This is a painless inflammatory muscle disease that results in muscle weakness. It is most commonly found in men aged 50 or over.

Neuromuscular disorders 2

1. H. Motor neurone disease
This is a neurological condition that targets the motor neurones and results in rapid deterioration of motor function in affected individuals.

2. J. Myasthenia gravis
Myasthenia gravis does not affect reflexes nor does it cause sensory loss, if either of these exist consider an alternative diagnosis.

3. E. Duchenne muscular dystrophy
This is a severe form of muscular dystrophy which affects mostly young boys. It is an X-linked recessive condition which is caused by a mutation in the gene for dystrophin, a protein which helps maintain a muscle fibre's cell membrane.

4. D. Charcot–Marie–Tooth disease
This is an inherited genetic condition which affects the peripheral nervous system (PNS). Patients commonly describe weakness in the hands and feet. Pes cavus and clawed toes are a common finding.

Vision loss 1

1. L. Retinitis pigmentosa
This condition typically presents as night blindness in childhood and adolescence. Typical fundoscopy examination findings are: attenuated retinal arterioles, a pale optic disc and bone spicule pigmentation.

2. G. Keratitis
Contact lens wearing is the main risk factor for bacterial keratitis. This is a sight threatening condition and must be treated promptly.

3. J. Primary open angle glaucoma
This condition classically results in optic disc cupping and loss of peripheral vision.

4. I. Posterior vitreous detachment
This occurs when the vitreous gel within the eye separates from the retina. Symptoms can include flashes and floaters in the affected eye.

5. D. Central retinal vein occlusion
This is caused by blockage of a retinal vein which results in fluid accumulation and blood leakage within the retina. On fundoscopy CRVO is described as having a "blood and thunder" appearance.

6. C. Central retinal artery occlusion
This patient has presented with classic features of CRAO, including sudden loss of vision which is painless and the appearance of a cherry red spot on fundoscopy.

Vision loss 2

1. A. Acute angle closure glaucoma
This condition is considered a medical emergency and results from closure of the angle between the iris and cornea. This closure causes a rapid elevation of intraocular pressure.

2. F. Iritis
In this condition there is inflammation of the iris, the coloured part of the eye. This condition is commonly associated with ankylosing spondylitis.

3. E. Giant cell arteritis
This condition affects the external carotid artery and associated branches, patients typically describe headache and jaw pain on the affected side. Visual loss can occur as a result of ischemia affecting the optic nerve.

4. H. Macular degeneration
Also known as age related macular degeneration (ARMD), this is a condition which may result in loss of vision.

5. B. Amaurosis fugax
This is a form of transient ischaemic attack (TIA).

6. K. Retinal detachment
This patient has a positive Shafer's sign which indicates a high likelihood that the retina has detached.

Women's and Sexual Health

5

AMENORRHOEA 1

A. Anorexia nervosa
B. Congenital adrenal hyperplasia
C. Cushing syndrome
D. Hypothyroidism
E. Kallmann syndrome
F. Menopause
G. Polycystic ovarian syndrome
H. Pregnancy
I. Primary ovarian insufficiency
J. Prolactinoma
K. Turner's syndrome

For each of the following, what is the MOST likely diagnosis?

1. A 16-year-old girl attends your clinic as she is concerned that she has not yet had her period. On examination she is 134 cm tall, has webbing of her neck and cubitus valgus. She has Tanner stage 1 breast and pubic hair development with shield chest and widely spaced nipples.

2. A 24-year-old barista presents with a 12-month history if amenorrhoea. She had menarche at age 13, has had erratic cycles since then occurring every two to three months with bleeds ranging from between three to seven days and varying amounts of flow. She has no significant medical history and takes no regular medication. On examination she has a BMI of 28, Tanner stage 4 breast and pubic hair development. You arrange for a transvaginal ultrasound which is unremarkable, she has an elevated FSH of 47 and a low sensitive oestradiol, you review her six weeks later and she has similar results.

3. A 22-year-old woman presents to your clinic with a delayed period. She explains that her periods are usually regular but reports that she is four weeks late. She has been feeling unwell for the past two weeks and reports that she has been

DOI: 10.1201/9781003459941-5

nauseated and has vomited several times a day, mostly in the morning, for the past three days. She is currently sexually active, reports that she has no significant past medical history and takes no regular medication.

4. A 25-year-old female presents with a six-month history of amenorrhoea, she explains that her periods have always been very erratic, occurring every two months or so. She recalls menarche at the age of 12. On examination she has acne across her cheeks and you note thick hair growth on her jaw line, she has a BMI of 28. You arrange for a transvaginal ultrasound is normal and she has a slightly elevated serum testosterone.

5. A 29-year-old woman presents with amenorrhoea for the past four months, she has recently noticed a one-month history of milky white discharge from bilateral nipples and reduced libido. Visual field examination reveals bitemporal hemianopia.

6. A 39-year-old woman presents for review, she is concerned that she has not had her period for the past 12 months. She also reports that she has gained 15 kg of weight during this period of time and has suffered from severe constipation. She has no significant past medical history. On examination you note that she is wearing excessive layers of clothing, has a BMI of 32, BP 136/88 mmHg, HR 52, has dry skin and thinning hair.

See page 135 for answers.

AMENORRHOEA 2

A. Anorexia nervosa
B. Congenital adrenal hyperplasia
C. Cushing syndrome
D. Hypothyroidism
E. Kallmann syndrome
F. Menopause
G. Polycystic ovarian syndrome
H. Pregnancy
I. Primary ovarian insufficiency
J. Prolactinoma
K. Turner's syndrome

For each of the following, what is the MOST likely diagnosis?

1. A 19-year-old female presents with primary amenorrhoea. She has no significant medical history and takes no regular medications. She is 156 cm tall and weighs 58 kg. On examination she has an enlarged clitoris, shallow vagina and excessive growth of facial and pubic hair. You arrange for laboratory testing

which reveals hypoglycaemia, hyponatraemia, hyperkalaemia and an elevated 17α-hydroxyprogesterone level.

2. A 21-year-old child care worker presents with amenorrhoea. She has never experienced menses. She has a past history significant for anosmia and takes no regular medication. On examination she has under developed secondary sexual characteristics with small breasts and a lack of both pubic and axillary hair. Pelvic examination reveals a shallow and narrow vagina with small labia minora.

3. A 16-year-old girl presents complaining of a several month history of nausea and vomiting. She tells you that she has been eating large volumes of food for the past three months and explains that after eating she vomits uncontrollably. On examination she has a BMI of 16. She has not had her period for the past three months and is currently sexually active with a single partner with whom she has been for one year.

4. A 23-year-old woman presents with secondary amenorrhoea, weight gain and increasing facial hair over the past 12 months. She had regular periods with 28-day cycles prior to this. On examination she has a BMI of 29, a blood pressure of 162/98 mmHg, a rounded and puffy face, violaceous striae affecting her lower abdomen and muscle wasting in her lower limbs.

5. A 41-year-old woman presents to your clinic complaining of a 14-month history of amenorrhoea. She has also been experiencing hot flushes for the past six months and night sweats. On examination she has a BMI of 30, Tanner stage 4 breast and pubic hair development.

See page 135 for answers.

BREAST PATHOLOGY 1

A. Breast abscess
B. Breast cyst
C. Breast lymphoma
D. Ductal carcinoma in situ
E. Ductal ectasia
F. Fat necrosis
G. Fibroadenoma
H. Galactocele
 I. Lactating adenoma
J. Mastitis
K. Nipple thrush
L. Nipple vasospasm
M. Mondor disease
N. Paget's disease of the breast
O. Papilloma
P. Phyllodes tumor

For each of the following, what is the MOST likely diagnosis?

1. A 32-year-old woman who is currently breastfeeding her 3-week-old child presents with left breast pain. She reports that the pain started two days ago and has gradually worsened. On examination she has a temperature of 38.3°C, her left breast is inflamed and tender to palpation without any obvious masses.

2. A 36-year-old woman presents with a seven-day history of right breast discomfort. You perform an examination of the affected breast and note a subcutaneous long and narrow red cord like lesion in the skin beneath the right breast which is more noticeable when the right arm is elevated.

3. A 27-year-old woman, who recently gave birth to a healthy girl, attends with a complaint of right sided breast lump. She noticed some changes in late pregnancy but has noticed the lump increasing in size over the past few weeks. She is currently breastfeeding. On examination you can palpate a right sided painless, mobile breast lump. An ultrasound is arranged which reveals a well circumscribed hypoechoic mass.

4. A 24-year-old woman presents to your clinic concerned about a lump she found in her breast while showering two weeks ago. On examination you palpate a small lump about 2 cm in diameter in her right breast. The lump is mobile within the breast tissue and moves away from beneath your fingers on firm palpation.

5. A 40-year-old woman presents with a three-month history of a lump in her left breast. On examination she has a mobile non tender lump, 10 cm in diameter, which is stretching the skin and creating a shiny appearance. The underlying veins are clearly visible and the skin appears as though it is about to ulcerate.

See page 136 for answers.

BREAST PATHOLOGY 2

A. **Breast abscess**
B. **Breast cyst**
C. **Breast lymphoma**
D. **Ductal carcinoma in situ**
E. **Ductal ectasia**
F. **Fat necrosis**
G. **Fibroadenoma**
H. **Galactocele**
I. **Lactating adenoma**
J. **Mastitis**
K. **Nipple thrush**
L. **Nipple vasospasm**
M. **Mondor disease**

N. Paget's disease of the breast
O. Papilloma
P. Phyllodes tumor

For each of the following, what is the MOST likely diagnosis?

1. A 58-year-old woman attends your clinic complaining of a three-month history of nipple discharge which is green-brown in colour. On examination you palpate a firm lump beneath the areola of her right breast, you also note nipple inversion.

2. A 56-year-old woman attends your clinic complaining of a lump in her right breast which she noticed three weeks ago, shortly after falling off her bike and injuring her chest. She has a history of subclinical hyperthyroidism and hypertension and takes perindopril on a regular basis. On examination she has a firm round lump in her right breast which is mildly tender.

3. A 24-year-old woman presents with left nipple pain. She is currently breast-feeding and explains that the pain is burning in nature and has been persistent for the past two days. She recently had a UTI and was treated with a course of antibiotics. She is otherwise on no regular medications. On examination she is afebrile, the left nipple is pink in colour and there is no palpable mass.

4. A 55-year-old librarian presents with a two-day history of right breast discomfort and swelling. She had silicone breast implant surgery two years ago. She has a past history of breast cancer which was successfully treated, she has also had bilateral mastectomy. On examination her right breast is swollen, tender to touch and firm. An ultrasound reveals fluid collection around the breast implant.

5. A 32-year-old woman presents to your clinic concerned about a lump she has found in her right breast. She noticed it yesterday while showering and reports that it is slightly tender to palpation. On examination she is tender in the right upper inner quadrant and you palpate a lump measuring 2 cm x 4 cm x 5 cm. You arrange for an ultrasound which reveals a well-defined anechoic lesion with posterior acoustic enhancement. You organise for needle aspiration which demonstrates a clear fluid, the lesion resolves after aspiration.

6. A 56-year-old woman attends for a routine check-up. She has been well and you perform a breast exam which is unremarkable. She is sent for a screening mammogram which reveals microcalcification within the breasts. You organise for a biopsy which reveals ducts distended by pleomorphic cells with central necrosis and no extension beyond the basement membrane.

See page 136 for answers.

BREAST PATHOLOGY 3

A. Breast abscess
B. Breast cyst
C. Breast lymphoma
D. Ductal carcinoma in situ
E. Ductal ectasia
F. Fat necrosis
G. Fibroadenoma
H. Galactocele
I. Lactating adenoma
J. Mastitis
K. Nipple thrush
L. Nipple vasospasm
M. Mondor disease
N. Paget's disease of the breast
O. Papilloma
P. Phyllodes tumor

For each of the following, what is the MOST likely diagnosis?

1. A 28-year-old woman presents with left sided breast pain for the past six days. She delivered a healthy child three months ago and is currently breastfeeding her. She explains that she noticed some redness in her breast six days ago and it slowly worsened. On examination she has erythema extending from the areola to the upper outer quadrant of the breast, you palpate an area of fluctuance 10 cm lateral to the areola on the left breast which is tender to touch.

2. A 58-year-old woman presents to your clinic with an itchy rash on her left breast. She first noticed it about four weeks ago and has seen another GP for it who prescribed topical corticosteroids. This treatment provided little relief. She has a history of subclinical hypothyroidism and takes no regular medications. On examination you note slight dimpling of the left nipple with overlying scaling which extends into the areola.

3. A 32-year-old woman attends your GP clinic concerned about a tender lump she has noticed beneath the areola of her left breast. She is currently breastfeeding her 6-month-old son. On palpation the lesion is 3 cm in diameter and feels cyst like.

4. A 25-year-old mother attends your clinic complaining of episodes of severe pain around her right nipple. She tells you that over the past few days she has been experiencing episodes of this lasting for a few seconds at a time, during these episodes the nipple turns white. She describes the pain as burning and throbbing in nature.

5. A 42-year-old woman presents complaining of blood-stained discharge from her left breast. Her paternal grandmother was diagnosed with breast cancer at

the age of 63 and she is very concerned about her presenting symptom. She has a history of anxiety and takes fluoxetine to help with this. She is a non-smoker and drinks alcohol on occasion. On examination there is a small of red coloured discharge from her left breast, you are not able to palpate a mass and she does not have palpable lymphadenopathy.

See pages 136–137 for answers.

MENSTRUAL IRREGULARITIES 1

A. Adenomyosis
B. Cervical ectropion
C. Dysfunctional uterine bleeding
D. Endometrial cancer
E. Endometriosis
F. Factor X deficiency
G. Hypothyroidism
H. Polycystic ovarian syndrome
 I. Uterine fibroid
 J. Uterine polyp
K. Von Willebrand disease

For each of the following, what is the MOST likely diagnosis?

1. A 25-year-old university student presents complaining of a three-month history of postcoital bleeding and intermenstrual bleeding. She has no significant medical history and takes no medication. You perform a speculum examination which reveals a reddish ring around the external os and a small amount of bleeding during examination.
2. A 22-year-old university student complains of a three-year history of irregular periods. She explains that her periods can be light at times and very heavy at others, there can also be up to two months between periods. On examination she has a BMI of 31, a normal abdominal and pelvic exam. You note thick and excessive facial hair. A transvaginal ultrasound reveals more than 20 follicles on the left ovary.
3. A 25-year-old woman presents with a 12-month history of menorrhagia. She reports that she has a 28-day cycle and bleeds heavily for six days, this is associated with some pain and cramping. You arrange for an ultrasound which reveals a well-defined, solid, concentric, hypoechoic uterine mass.
4. A 65-year-old woman attends your clinic with an episode of postmenopausal bleeding which has lasted for the past five days.
5. A 34-year-old woman complains of a five-year history of lower abdominal pain associated with heavy menstrual bleeds. She and her partner have been trying

to conceive without success for the past 12 months. She is referred to a gynae-cologist and a laparoscopy is performed to assess tubal patency, a chocolate-coloured cyst is found on her right ovary.

6. A 31-year-old woman presents with a long history of heavy menstrual bleeds. She suffers from migraines for which she takes ibuprofen and Panadol almost daily and has done this for the past 12 months. Since commencing this treatment, she reports that her periods have become heavier and she has also been experiencing epistaxis which can take some time to resolve. She explains that her father has a history of prolonged nose bleeds. You arrange for some blood tests which reveal normal PT and an increased PTT.

See page 137 for answers.

MENSTRUAL IRREGULARITIES 2

A. **Adenomyosis**
B. **Cervical ectropion**
C. **Dysfunctional uterine bleeding**
D. **Endometrial cancer**
E. **Endometriosis**
F. **Factor X deficiency**
G. **Hypothyroidism**
H. **Polycystic ovarian syndrome**
I. **Uterine Fibroid**
J. **Uterine Polyp**
K. **Von Willebrand disease**

For each of the following, what is the MOST likely diagnosis?

1. A 36-year-old woman presents to your GP clinic complaining of heavy menstrual bleeding for the past eight months. She also complains of intermenstrual bleeds during this time. Abdominal examination and internal examination are unremarkable. You arrange for an ultrasound which reveals a focal echogenic, round lesion disrupting the normal echotexture of the endometrium.

2. A 26-year-old woman attends your clinic complaining of a 16-month history of heavy menstrual periods. She has no significant past medical history and takes no regular medication. Physical examination reveals multiple bruises across her lower limbs and abdomen, she tells you that she bruises easily and finds it hard to stop small cuts from bleeding.

3. A 49-year-old G3P3 woman attends your clinic complaining of an 18-month history of menorrhagia and dysmenorrhoea. She reports that she has a 28-day cycle with four days of bleeding but they now occur more frequently at 23 days. She explains that she bleeds heavily on the first three days of every cycle, has

to change her pads every few hours and has to use tampons also. She has no other symptoms, has no significant medical history and does not use any regular medications. On examination she has a uniformly enlarged uterus which is boggy, tender and freely motile. Urine HCG is negative.

4. A 42-year-old woman presents to your clinic with a five-month history of irregular and heavy periods. Her last period ended seven days ago and lasted for nine days, the period prior to this was two months ago and lasted for five days. She explains that she has had to use multiple overnight pads during menses, she normally uses tampons alone. Prior to this her periods were regular with a 28-day cycle and five days of bleeding. Physical examination reveals no abnormality. She has a negative urine pregnancy test and her pelvic ultrasound is normal.

5. A 38-year-old woman presents with a two-year history of menorrhagia. She explains that she has been very fatigued, has had severe constipation and has had some weight gain during this time. On examination she is afebrile, has a heart rate of 56 which is regular and has thinning of her hair. Her abdominal and internal examination findings are normal.

See pages 137–138 for answers.

MALE INFERTILITY 1

A. Cryptorchidism
B. Del Castillo syndrome
C. Drug induced infertility
D. Hyperprolactinaemia
E. Kallmann syndrome
F. Klinefelter syndrome
G. Primary ciliary dyskinesia
H. Varicocele
I. Young's syndrome

For each of the following, what is the MOST likely diagnosis?

1. A 31-year-old male attends your clinic with his partner, they have been trying to conceive for the past 17 months without any success. The female partner has been assessed and found to not have any cause for infertility. He has no significant medical history and takes no regular medication. You examine his scrotum and find that the left hemi-scrotum rests lower than the right. Palpation of the left side feels like a bag of worms.

2. A 32-year-old welder presents with a 12-month history of infertility. His current partner has children from another marriage. He has no significant history and takes no regular medication. On examination he has well developed secondary sexual characteristics, examination of his testes and

penis is unremarkable. Investigations reveal normal LH, FSH and testosterone levels. You arrange for a testicular biopsy which reveals that the seminiferous tubules contain Sertoli cells alone with absence of germ cells.

3. A 38-year-old male presents complaining of infertility. He has been in a relationship with his current partner for the past 18 months and for the past eight months they have been trying to conceive without success. He suffers from a mild intellectual disability but otherwise has no significant medical history and takes no regular medication. On examination he is 198 cm tall, lacks facial hair, has bilateral gynaecomastia and has small testes.

4. A 27-year-old man presents to your clinic complaining of a nine-month history of infertility. He has a history of psoriasis and depression but takes no regular medication. On examination he has under developed secondary sexual characteristics, a small penis and sparse pubic hair (Tanner stage 2). You note that he has a reduced sense of smell but cranial nerve examination is otherwise well.

See page 138 for answers.

MALE INFERTILITY 2

A. **Cryptorchidism**
B. **Del Castillo syndrome**
C. **Drug induced infertility**
D. **Hyperprolactinaemia**
E. **Kallmann syndrome**
F. **Klinefelter syndrome**
G. **Primary ciliary dyskinesia**
H. **Varicocele**
I. **Young's syndrome**

For each of the following, what is the MOST likely diagnosis?

1. A 31-year-old male presents to your clinic complaining of infertility for the past 12 months. His partner has previously had children in another relationship. He has a long history of recurrent nasal congestion and productive cough. You arranged for imaging six months ago which revealed bronchiectasis, dextrocardia and situs inversus.

2. A 28-year-old architect presents with his partner after 12 months of failure to conceive. He has a history of hypertension and hyperlipidaemia. He is currently using simvastatin and captopril. On examination he has secondary sexual characteristics appropriate for his age. Semen analysis reveals a complete lack of sperm. FSH and testosterone levels are within normal range. You arrange for an

ultrasound of his testes which are not found to be present within his scrotum or his inguinal canals.

3. A 26-year-old male presents to your clinic with a complaint of primary infertility. He and his partner have been trying to conceive for the past 11 months without success, she has been reviewed by her gynaecologist and not found to have any cause for infertility. He has a long history of recurrent chest infections and rhinosinusitis otherwise he is well. You arrange for sperm analysis which reveals an absence of spermatozoa, biopsy of the testes reveals normal spermatogenesis.

4. A 30-year-old bodybuilder presents to your clinic after 19 months of failure to conceive. His wife was seen by a gynaecologist and was found to have no fertility problems. He has a past history of subcoronal hypospadias (which was surgically corrected at 18 months of age), depression and severe acne. He takes no regular medication, he had previously been on long term anabolic steroids for physique and performance enhancing purposes, he stopped using these 12 months ago. On examination he has well developed secondary sexual characteristics. FSH, LH and testosterone were found to be low.

5. A 37-year-old male presents to your clinic complaining of reduced libido, he tells you that he and his partner have been trying to conceive for the past 18 months without success. He reports that he has been suffering from chronic headaches for the past two years and has been taking Panadol to help with this, he has no other significant medical history. On examination he has well developed secondary sexual characteristics, he has bitemporal hemianopia on visual examination. Investigations reveal reduced LH, FSH and testosterone.

See page 138 for answers.

COMPLICATIONS OF PREGNANCY 1

A. Blighted ovum
B. Chorioamnionitis
C. Complete miscarriage
D. Cornual pregnancy
E. Hydatidiform mole
F. Inevitable miscarriage
G. Missed miscarriage
H. Recurrent miscarriage
I. Threatened miscarriage

For each of the following, what is the MOST likely diagnosis?

1. A 26-year-old primigravid woman presents for review at 12 weeks. She complains of a brown coloured discharge over the past few days and explains that while she had severe nausea and vomiting a few weeks ago these symptoms have now settled. You arrange for an ultrasound which reveals a fetus with an absent heartbeat.

2. A 30-year-old woman presents to your GP clinic with a seven-week history of amenorrhoea. She has a positive urine pregnancy test. You arrange for an ultrasound which reveals a gestational sac which corresponds to a gestational age of 7 weeks and 1 day. A yolk sac is visible but you cannot identify an embryo.

3. A 26-year-old primigravid woman attends your emergency department with per vaginal bleeding. She is currently 13 weeks' gestation. Ultrasound reveals multiple cystic spaces within the uterus that resemble a "bunch of grapes".

4. A 28-year-old woman who is 22 weeks' gestation presents with a fever, lower abdominal discomfort and foul-smelling vaginal discharge. On examination she has a temperature of 38.7°C, heart rate 106 and a respiratory rate 20. Her abdomen is tender in the suprapubic region and speculum examination reveals a dilated cervix with discharge of fluid.

5. A 33-year-old woman presents at 19 weeks' gestation. She complains of vaginal bleeding and lower abdominal pain. On examination she has a temperature of 36.8°C, heart rate 88, respiratory rate 18. Her abdomen is tender in the suprapubic region, internal exam reveals a closed cervix.

See page 139 for answers.

COMPLICATIONS OF PREGNANCY 2

A. Blighted ovum
B. Chorioamnionitis
C. Complete miscarriage
D. Cornual pregnancy
E. Hydatidiform mole
F. Inevitable miscarriage
G. Missed miscarriage
H. Recurrent miscarriage
I. Threatened miscarriage

For each of the following, what is the MOST likely diagnosis?

1. A 25-year-old woman presents at 11 weeks' gestation. She complains of heavy vaginal bleeding, passage of clots and lower abdominal pain. On examination she has a temperature of 36.6°C, heart rate 72, respiratory rate 20. Her abdomen is tender in the suprapubic region, internal exam reveals a partially open cervix.

2. Lidia a 22-year-old woman is 10 weeks' gestation and attends your emergency department complaining of abdominal cramping since this morning, she went to the bathroom and passed a large clot. She has been bleeding since this episode. Her last ultrasound was performed at six weeks which showed an intra-uterine pregnancy. You arrange for an ultrasound in your department which reveals an empty uterus.

3. A 28-year-old woman your emergency with left sided abdominal pain. You perform a urine HCG which is positive. Ultrasound reveals implantation in the left horn of the uterus.

4. A 29-year-old woman who is ten weeks pregnant presents to your clinic complaining of PV bleeding. An ultrasound is arranged which confirms a silent miscarriage. She is very distressed and explains that she has seen another GP in the past and has had miscarriages at ten and 12 weeks respectively over the past 18 months.

See page 139 for answers.

VULVOVAGINAL PATHOLOGY 1

A. Allergic contact dermatitis
B. Atrophic vaginitis
C. Bartholin's cyst
D. Condyloma acuminata
E. Folliculitis
F. Fox–Fordyce disease
G. Lichen sclerosus
H. Lichen planus
I. Molluscum contagiosum
J. Psoriasis
K. Skene's duct cyst
L. Vulvovaginal candidiasis

For each of the following, what is the MOST likely diagnosis?

1. A 65-year-old attends your clinic complaining of vulvar itch. Her symptoms have been present for six months. She is concerned as she has a new sexual partner and has found sexual penetration very painful. On examination you note that the skin of the vulva is thinned and pale in colour. You also note loss of the left labia minora and that the hood of the clitoris is retracted.

2. A 28-year-old woman presents to your clinic complaining of a three-week history of genital itch and discomfort. On examination there is a well demarcated, symmetrical, silver, scaly plaque overlying bilateral labia majora.

3. A 35-year-old woman presents complaining of a tender lump in her right labia majora. She reports she has had painless swelling for the past six months but the pain has been present for the past two days and the swelling has slowly worsened. On examination there is a fluctuant, large and tender lump involving the right labia majora and vagina. The lump is located in the posterolateral inferior third of the vagina, appears shiny has some purulent discharge from an opening in its surface. It measures 5 cm long and 3 cm wide.

4. A 23-year-old woman presents to your clinic for review of an itchy rash she has developed over the past 24 hours. She reports that she first noticed the rash yesterday while changing her menstrual pad. On examination there are two well circumscribed erythematous lesions which are asymmetrical over the left labia majora, you note scratch marks in the skin. She explains that she is visiting from interstate and her menses started three days ago. She had not planned for it and had to use a brand of pads she normally does not use as they were the only type available at the local shop.

See page 139 for answers.

VULVOVAGINAL PATHOLOGY 2

A. **Allergic contact dermatitis**
B. **Atrophic vaginitis**
C. **Bartholin's cyst**
D. **Condyloma acuminata**
E. **Folliculitis**
F. **Fox–Fordyce disease**
G. **Lichen sclerosus**
H. **Lichen planus**
I. **Molluscum contagiosum**
J. **Psoriasis**
K. **Skene's duct cyst**
L. **Vulvovaginal candidiasis**

For each of the following, what is the MOST likely diagnosis?

1. A 25-year-old retail worker attends your metropolitan GP clinic for review. She complains of itch around her vulva of several weeks duration and she has noticed some small bumps in her skin. On examination you find wart like growths over the labia minora on the right side.

2. A 25-year-old woman presents to your clinic complaining of vaginal itch, dysuria and dyspareunia. She reports that there has not been any associated vaginal bleeding. She gave birth six months ago and is currently breast

feeding. She had an uncomplicated pregnancy and has no significant medical history.

3. A 23-year-old woman presents with a two-week history of vulvar itch. Over the past five days she has had white curdy vaginal discharge. On examination she has erythema and swelling of the vulva.

4. A 53-year-old woman presents to your country practice complaining of an itchy rash. She tells you that she is itchy around her lower abdomen, her buttocks and particularly in her groin region. She was out with friends two nights ago and spent some time in a hot tub. On examination you note papules and pustules in the areas of concern.

5. A 31-year-old woman presents with a rash. She explains that she has a few bumps in her skin around the vulva. She noticed them a few weeks ago and reports that they are painless and are increasing in number. On examination you find multiple skin-coloured bumps in the area of concern with dimples in their centres. They have a pearl like appearance.

See page 140 for answers.

FEMALE INFERTILITY 1

A. Asherman's syndrome
B. Cushing's disease
C. Endometriosis
D. Fallopian tube damage
E. Hashimoto's thyroiditis
F. Hyperprolactinaemia
G. Hypogonadotrophic hypogonadism
H. Polycystic ovarian syndrome
I. Premature ovarian failure
J. Uterine fibroid

For each of the following, what is the MOST likely diagnosis?

1. A 21-year-old woman presents complaining of infertility, she and her partner have been trying to conceive naturally for the past 12 months without success. She explains that she has never really had a regular cycle, her periods are infrequent and occur every two to three months. Examination reveals pubic hair and breast development at Tanner stage 2. Investigation reveals low FSH, LH and serum oestradiol.

2. A 34-year-old woman explains that she has been trying to fall pregnant with her partner for the past nine months without success. Samantha has gained 7 kg in this time, reports that she has noticed excess hair growth in her axillae and across her face, her periods have become very irregular and she explains that

she has been feeling very down. Investigations reveal high cortisol and high ACTH levels.

3. A 32-year-old woman presents complaining of a two-year history of menorrhagia and infertility. She reports that her periods are regular and that she has a 28-day cycle but over this period of time she has had much heavier and longer episodes of bleeding. Previously she bled for five days every cycle and could get through her bleeds with the use of tampons alone, she now reports that her bleeds last for up to seven days and she has to use overnight pads and tampons. She experiences some pain prior to and during menses which she manages with NSAIDs. You perform a bimanual examination which reveals a bulky uterus.

4. A 27-year-old accountant presents complaining of a one-year history of amenorrhoea. She has no significant past medical history and does not use any regular medications. She explains that prior to this her periods were quite erratic, she had menarche at the age of 14 and tells you that her cycles lasted anywhere between one and three months in duration and explains that the duration and amount of bleeding were quite variable. She has a regular sexual partner and they have been trying to conceive for the past six months naturally without success. On examination she has a BMI of 23, BP of 122/86 mmHg, soft and nontender abdomen, she also has an unremarkable breast and pelvic examination. She has a random BSL of 7.4, FSH of 48 IU and a low sensitive oestradiol. You repeat the investigations four weeks later and find similar results.

See page 140 for answers.

FEMALE INFERTILITY 2

A. **Asherman's syndrome**
B. **Cushing's disease**
C. **Endometriosis**
D. **Fallopian tube damage**
E. **Hashimoto's thyroiditis**
F. **Hyperprolactinaemia**
G. **Hypogonadotrophic hypogonadism**
H. **Polycystic ovarian syndrome**
I. **Premature ovarian failure**
J. **Uterine fibroid**

For each of the following, what is the MOST likely diagnosis?

1. A 32-year-old woman has a 12-month complaint of worsening fatigue, constipation and hair loss. She further explains that she and her partner have tried to conceive over this period of time without success. She has a history of vitiligo

since the age of 20 and no other significant past medical history. Investigations reveal that she is TPO positive.

2. A 25-year-old woman presents complaining of infertility. She and her partner have been trying to conceive naturally for the past 12 months. She reports that she has been having irregular periods, they occur every two to three months. She has no significant past medical history and takes no regular medications. On examination she has acne across her face and you note that she has a significant amount of facial hair on her upper lip and a BMI of 28.

3. A 33-year-old G1P1 woman presents to your clinic complaining of infertility. She and her partner have been trying to conceive for the past 12 months. She reports that her periods have been much lighter since the birth of her now 18-month-old son. Her son was delivered by caesarean section and the delivery was complicated by endometritis. You arrange for a hysteroscopy which reveals intra-uterine adhesions.

4. A 22-year-old woman presents to your GP clinic with an 18-month history of painful periods, difficulties conceiving for the past 12 months and painful intercourse. You send her for specialist review and she subsequently has a laparoscopy which reveals chocolate cysts affecting her ovaries bilaterally, there are also red dots across the pelvic walls and fallopian tubes.

5. A 32-year-old woman presents to your clinic complaining of a four-month history of headache. She explains that she had her last period just prior to onset of these symptoms and has a reduced sex drive. Physical examination reveals that she has bitemporal hemianopia.

See pages 140–141 for answers.

OBSTETRIC COMPLICATIONS 1

A. Amniotic fluid embolism
B. Eclampsia
C. Ectopic pregnancy
D. HELLP syndrome
E. Placental abruption
F. Placenta praevia
G. Postpartum haemorrhage
H. Pre-Eclampsia
 I. Preterm premature rupture of membranes
J. Prolapsed umbilical cord
K. Shoulder dystocia
L. Uterus inversion
M. Uterus rupture

For each of the following, what is the MOST likely diagnosis?

1. A 29-year-old G1P0 woman presents to your emergency department concerned as she believes her waters have broken. She is 36 weeks' gestation; she has had an uncomplicated pregnancy until now. She has not experienced any contractions. She has no significant medical history and takes no regular medication. She is a smoker and has smoked two cigarettes a day throughout her pregnancy. You perform a sterile speculum examination which reveals a closed cervix and a pool of fluid within the vagina. Nitrazine paper test is performed, this turns blue.

2. A 29-year-old pregnant woman, G2P1, presents to your rural emergency department complaining of a severe headache, she tells you that it affects most of her head. She has had some Panadol throughout the day but has found little relief. She is currently 35 weeks' gestation. She took her blood pressure this morning at the local pharmacy and had a reading of 168/96 mmHg, The pharmacist advised her to present to your emergency department. You take her blood pressure, which reads 160/98 mmHg. You perform a urine dipstick which reveals proteinuria 3+. Suddenly she drops to the floor, loses consciousness, her body stiffens up and she begins to jerk uncontrollably.

3. A 26-year-old pregnant woman, G1P0, presents to your clinic complaining of a two-day history of headache, she explains that it is generalised and mildly uncomfortable. She is currently 26 weeks' gestation. She took her blood pressure last night at home on her father's blood pressure device and had a reading of 164/92 mmHg, she thought the elevation may have been due to anxiety and the pain of the headache. She decided to sleep on it and see you in the morning. You take her blood pressure today which reads 167/93 mmHg. Her last reading two weeks ago was 120/84. You perform a urine dipstick which reveals proteinuria 2+.

4. A 30-year-old G2P1 woman presents to your emergency department with vaginal bleeding. She is currently 35 weeks' gestation. She tells you that she has had uterine contractions which started a few hours ago and have been happening every one to two minutes for the past hour. She is a smoker and smokes 20 cigarettes a day. She has no other significant medical history and takes no regular medication. On examination she has a BP of 158/72 mmHg, heart rate of 108 bpm and a temperature of 36.5°C. She has a firm, tender uterus and she has dark blood exiting her vagina. The fetal heart rate is 162 bpm. Digital cervical examination reveals a cervix which is 8 cm dilated.

5. A 29-year-old G2P1 woman attends her local hospital in labour. She is 38 weeks' gestation; she has had an uneventful pregnancy. She has a history of recurrent urinary tract infections and an appendicectomy, she takes no regular medication. She delivers a healthy child after a six-hour labour. Shortly after delivery of her placenta she becomes short of breath, develops vaginal bleeding and loses consciousness. On examination she has a BP of 75/42 mmHg, HR 112 beats per minute, RR of 26 breaths per minute and a temperature of 36.7°C.

See page 141 for answers.

OBSTETRIC COMPLICATIONS 2

A. **Amniotic fluid embolism**
B. **Eclampsia**
C. **Ectopic pregnancy**
D. **HELLP syndrome**
E. **Placental abruption**
F. **Placenta praevia**
G. **Postpartum haemorrhage**
H. **Pre-Eclampsia**
I. **Preterm premature rupture of membranes**
J. **Prolapsed umbilical cord**
K. **Shoulder dystocia**
L. **Uterus inversion**
M. **Uterus rupture**

For each of the following, what is the MOST likely diagnosis?

1. A 26-year-old G1P0 woman presents in labour to your local hospital. She is currently 39 weeks' gestation and has been managed for gestational diabetes mellitus during her pregnancy. On examination her cervix is fully dilated and she is in the second stage of delivery. An hour after her presentation the fetal head is delivered with external rotation. Turtle sign quickly follows the delivery of the head.

2. A 23-year-old woman attends your emergency department with severe left sided abdominal pain associated with vaginal bleeding and cramping. Her symptoms started an hour ago and have progressively worsened. On examination she is tender in her left iliac fossa, she has a BP of 98/72 mmHg, heart rate of 108 bpm. Speculum examination is unremarkable. You arrange for bloods which reveal an Hb of 87 and a beta-HCG of 1700. You arrange for a pelvic ultrasound which reveals an empty uterus.

3. A 30-year-old woman presents to your emergency department via ambulance after a home birth. She started passing a lot of blood an hour after delivery of a healthy child. She has no significant past medical history and takes no regular medications. Other than hyperemesis she has had an uneventful pregnancy. On examination she has a BP of 82/56 mmHg, HR 120 beats per minute, RR of 18 breaths per minute and a temperature of 36.7°C. Her uterus is enlarged and soft.

4. A 28-year-old pregnant woman, G2P1, presents to your emergency department with sudden heavy vaginal bleeding. She is currently 34 weeks' gestation and she has not had any antenatal care or follow up with her local health services during her pregnancy. She denies any pain. She has no significant past medical history and takes no regular medications. On examination her observations

are within normal limits, her abdomen and uterus are non-tender on palpation. CTG findings are normal.

5. A 31-year-old G2P1 woman presents to your labour ward. She is 40 weeks' gestation and has had an uneventful pregnancy. On examination she is 8 cm dilated and her membranes are intact she has a BP of 122/80 mmHg, HR 78 beats per minute, RR of 18 breaths per minute and a temperature of 36.7°C. Fetal heart rate is 138 without decelerations. Shortly after arrival her waters break, her pain level increases significantly. You note prolonged decelerations and fetal heart rate begins to decrease. You perform an examination; her cervix is now at 10 cm and you palpate a pulsatile umbilical cord.

See pages 141–142 for answers.

DYSMENORRHOEA

A. **Adenomyosis**
B. **Adhesions**
C. **Cervical stenosis**
D. **Ectopic pregnancy**
E. **Endometriosis**
F. **Fibroids**
G. **Hematometra**
H. **Miscarriage**
 I. **Ovarian carcinoma**
J. **Pelvic inflammatory disease**
K. **Uterine hypoplasia**

For each of the following, what is the MOST likely diagnosis?

1. A 31-year-old woman presents with an 18-month history of dysmenorrhoea and menorrhagia. She explains that her cycles are very regular and last 30 days. She bleeds heavily for the about five to six days and reports that she has significant discomfort for three days prior to and the first couple days of her period. You arrange for an ultrasound which reveals a well-defined, solid, concentric, hypoechoic uterine mass.

2. A 30-year-old woman presents to your GP clinic complaining of a three-year history of dysmenorrhoea and menorrhagia. She has been trying to conceive for the past 18 months without success. Over the past four months she has developed lower abdominal pain radiating into her rectum. On rectovaginal examination you palpate small nodules which are significantly tender. You refer her to a gynaecologist who arranges for a laparoscopy, chocolate-coloured cysts are found on bilateral ovaries and fallopian tubes.

3. A 36-year-old woman presents to your GP clinic complaining of a six-month history of dysmenorrhoea and amenorrhoea for the past two months. Her periods are usually very regular and she has a 28-day cycle. She has been pregnant twice and has delivered two healthy children aged five and three years via vaginal deliveries without complication. She has had a LLETZ procedure for CIN 2 changes seven months ago. On examination she has lower abdominal discomfort and a boggy uterus on palpation. Speculum examination reveals an occluded cervix. Urine HCG is negative.

4. A 23-year-old woman presents with a two-day history of pelvic pain and heavy menstrual bleeding. She reports that she has been suffering from dyspareunia for the past four days and has had offensive vaginal discharge during this period of time. On examination she has cervical motion tenderness. She has been with her current sexual partner for the past two months.

5. A 23-year-old interior designer presents to your emergency department with abdominal discomfort and vaginal bleeding. Her symptoms started four hours ago, she normally has cramping and pain during menses but this feels worse than her regular period. On examination she appears pale and distressed. She has a rigid abdomen, has a temperature of 36.7°C, heart rate of 116 beats per minute and a BP of 110/75 mmHg. She has a positive urine HCG and a bedside USS reveals an empty uterus.

See page 142 for answers.

SEXUALLY TRANSMITTED INFECTION 1

A. **Bacterial vaginosis**
B. **Candidiasis**
C. **Chlamydia trachomatis**
D. **Donovanosis**
E. **Genital herpes**
F. **Gonorrhoea**
G. **Human papillomavirus**
H. **Lymphogranuloma venerum**
I. **Syphilis**
J. **Trichomoniasis**

For each of the following, what is the MOST likely diagnosis?

1. A 28-year-old secretary presents to your clinic concerned about vaginal discharge and irritation for the past four days. She reports that the small amount of discharge she has is clear and non-offensive, she has no associated bleeding. She has had three sexual partners in the past year and has been with her current

partner for at least three months. On vaginal examination you note that her cervix bled easily upon swabbing, you also note the presence of Mirena strings.

2. A 39-year-old lady attends your clinic complaining of a six-day history of vaginal discharge that she describes as having an offensive fishy odour. On physical examination, you note a grey coloured offensive discharge.

3. A 19-year-old university student presents for review at her university health service. She complains of itch around her vulva of several weeks duration and she has noticed some small bumps in her skin. The bumps are causing her much grief and she would like to know what she can do to treat them. On examination you find wart like growths over the labia minora on the right side.

4. A 31-year-old woman attends for her routine antenatal visit, she is currently in the second trimester of her first pregnancy. On review she is concerned about a painful ulceration over her left labia majora. Examination reveals a cluster of vesicles on the skin over her left labia majora associated with inguinal lymph node enlargement on the same side.

See pages 142–143 for answers.

SEXUALLY TRANSMITTED INFECTION 2

A. Bacterial vaginosis
B. Candidiasis
C. Chlamydia trachomatis
D. Donovanosis
E. Genital herpes
F. Gonorrhoea
G. Human papillomavirus
H. Lymphogranuloma venerum
I. Syphilis
J. Trichomoniasis

For each of the following, what is the MOST likely diagnosis?

1. A 23-year-old receptionist presents to your busy city clinic with a history of vaginal itch, malodour and profuse frothy discharge for the past two weeks. She reports a single male sexual partner who is asymptomatic. On speculum examination you note a strawberry cervix.

2. A 23-year-old male attends your clinic complaining of dysuria for the past two days. He reports a thick yellow coloured urethral discharge associated with this and testicular tenderness. On examination he has a temperature of 37.7°C, you note a thick yellow discharge at the urethral meatus and tenderness on palpation of red, swollen testes bilaterally.

3. A 32-year-old lady presents to you with a three-day history of dysuria associated with vaginal itch. Speculum examination of the vagina reveals a foul smelling thick white discharge with a "cottage cheese" appearance.

4. A 24-year-old carpenter attends your surgery complaining of a sore on his penis. The sore is painless and he noticed it two days ago. He has had multiple male partners over the past 12 months and is regularly involved in casual sex with unknown males. Examination reveals a round lesion on the shaft of his penis and inguinal lymph node enlargement in bilateral groins. An EIA is initially requested and this returns reactive, a diagnosis is subsequently confirmed with a positive RPR.

See page 143 for answers.

GENETIC DISORDERS 1

A. Angelman syndrome
B. Down syndrome (Trisomy 21)
C. Edwards syndrome (Trisomy 18)
D. Fragile X syndrome
E. Klinefelter syndrome (XXY)
F. Marfan syndrome
G. Noonan syndrome
H. Patau syndrome (Trisomy 13)
 I. Turner syndrome
J. Williams syndrome

For each of the following, what is the MOST likely diagnosis?

1. A 32-year-old caucasian female presents to your GP clinic complaining of a three-day history of central chest pain associated with exertion. She explains that the pain radiates to her back and can be quite severe. She has a past medical history significant for bilateral cataract surgery and chronic lumbar back pain. She has a family history significant for "heart issues", her father passed away suddenly as a result of this condition at the age of 36. On examination she has elongated arms, pectus excavatum and you note a diastolic murmur over the aortic area.

2. A 41-year-old woman presents to your obstetrics ward in labour. She lives in a remote community and has not been able to attend antenatal visits during her pregnancy. She has no significant medical history nor does she take any regular medications. She gives birth to a baby boy. On examination at birth, he is noted to have hypotonia, a flat rounded face with small eyes, nose and mouth. You also note a slightly bent fifth digit in his left hand.

3. A 43-year-old G2P2 woman presents to your clinic with her newborn daughter for her 6-week newborn check. She has been feeding poorly in recent weeks

and suffers from severe episodes of infantile colic. On examination she has elfin like facial features, a broad forehead, microcephaly and a wide mouth. Cardiac exam reveals a systolic murmur and on abdominal examination you note a small umbilical hernia.

4. A 12-year-old male presents to your clinic with his mother who is concerned about learning difficulties at school. He has fallen behind in his class and his mother has been called into the school on several occasions to discuss his poor performance. He has had a long history of learning difficulties since commencing primary school. He was born at term, he has no significant past medical history, he takes no regular medications and his immunisations are current. On examination you note a long face, protruding ears and macro-orchidism.

See page 143 for answers.

GENETIC DISORDERS 2

A. **Angelman syndrome**
B. **Down syndrome (Trisomy 21)**
C. **Edwards syndrome (Trisomy 18)**
D. **Fragile X syndrome**
E. **Klinefelter syndrome (XXY)**
F. **Marfan syndrome**
G. **Noonan syndrome**
H. **Patau syndrome (Trisomy 13)**
I. **Turner syndrome**
J. **Williams syndrome**

For each of the following, what is the MOST likely diagnosis?

1. A 1-year-old boy presents with his mother who is concerned about delayed development and constipation. He has a history of pulmonary stenosis and undescended testicles which have been surgically repaired. Physical examination reveals low set ears and antimongoloid palpebral slant.

2. A 29-year-old male presents with his partner complaining of a 24-month history of infertility. He has no significant past medical history and takes no regular medications. He is 190 cm tall, 87 kg and has noticeable gynaecomastia. On genital examination he has small testes with a volume < 4 ml (normal range 5–15 ml).

3. A 15-year-old girl attends your clinic with her mother who is concerned that she has not yet had her period. On examination she is 122 cm tall, has webbing of her neck and cubitus valgus. She has no breast development with shield chest and widely spaced nipples. You also note that she has no visible pubic or axillary hair.

4. A 7-year-old boy is referred to your paediatric clinic for developmental delay and learning difficulties. From birth he has had a near absence of speech and has a five-year history of tonic clonic seizures. On examination he has a sunken nasal bridge, mandibular protrusion and appears to be smiling and laughing.

See pages 143–144 for answers.

PELVIC-ABDOMINAL PAIN 1

A. Adenomyosis
B. Appendicitis
C. Endometriosis
D. Endometritis
E. Mittelschmerz
F. Ovarian hyperstimulation syndrome
G. Ovarian torsion
H. Pelvic inflammatory disease
I. Pyelonephritis
J. Renal calculus
K. Ruptured ectopic pregnancy
L. Ruptured ovarian cyst

For each of the following, what is the MOST likely diagnosis?

1. A 26-year-old woman presents to your emergency department with severe left iliac fossa pain. The pain started about three hours ago and she describes it as the worst pain she has felt. She cannot recall her last period and takes no regular medication. On examination she appears pale and distressed. She has a rigid abdomen, has a temperature of 36.1°C, heart rate of 121 beats per minute and a BP of 86/62 mmHg. She has a positive urine HCG and a bedside USS reveals an empty uterus.

2. A 25-year-old woman presents with right iliac fossa pain. Her pain started today and was of sudden onset. She tells you her last period was about two weeks ago. On examination she has a temperature of 36.1°C and tenderness in her right lower abdomen.

3. A 23-year-old university student is brought into your emergency department complaining of severe pelvic pain. Her symptoms started an hour after having sexual intercourse with her boyfriend. She has no significant medical history. On examination she has a temperature of 36.7°C, heart rate of 89 beats per minute and a BP of 116/82 mmHg. She is tender on palpation of the right iliac fossa. You perform a urine HCG test which is negative. Ultrasound exam reveals fluid around the right ovary and within the pouch of Douglas. There is also a cystic mass seen on the right ovary measuring 3 cm x 4 cm.

4. A 24-year-old woman attends your clinic complaining of a one-day history of abdominal pain associated with nausea and multiple episodes of vomiting. She reports that the pain started last night and has gradually worsened. The pain is around her belly button and dull in nature. Her last menstrual period was two weeks ago. On examination she has a temperature of 38.1°C and rebound tenderness in her right lower abdomen.

5. A 26-year-old woman presents to your emergency department complaining of pelvic pain and per vaginal bleeding. She had a surgical abortion five days ago. On examination she has a temperature of 37.9°C and suprapubic tenderness on palpation.

See page 144 for answers.

PELVIC-ABDOMINAL PAIN 2

A. **Adenomyosis**
B. **Appendicitis**
C. **Endometriosis**
D. **Endometritis**
E. **Mittelschmerz**
F. **Ovarian hyperstimulation syndrome**
G. **Ovarian torsion**
H. **Pelvic inflammatory disease**
 I. **Pyelonephritis**
 J. **Renal calculus**
K. **Ruptured ectopic pregnancy**
L. **Ruptured ovarian cyst**

For each of the following, what is the MOST likely diagnosis?

1. A 32-year-old woman presents with severe abdominal pain and multiple episodes of vomiting. She is currently undergoing IVF treatment and has no significant past medical history. On examination there is shifting dullness. She takes no regular medications.

2. A 31-year-old woman presents to your practice with a complaint of dysmenorrhoea. Her symptoms have been present for the past six months. Over the past two months she has developed lower abdominal pain radiating into her rectum and suffers from dyspareunia. She has been trying to conceive with her partner for the past 12 months without success, she has no other significant medical history. On rectovaginal examination you palpate small nodules which are significantly tender.

3. A 20-year-old woman presents to your metropolitan emergency department with severe abdominal pain. She explains that her symptoms started six hours

ago, initially the pain was intermittent but is now constant, severe and mostly on the right side. Prior to attending your department, she vomited four times at home. On examination she is extremely tender in the right iliac fossa. She has a negative urine HCG. You arrange for an ultrasound which reveals a swollen right ovary, free pelvic fluid and a positive follicular ring sign.

4. A 34-year-old woman presents with a two-hour history of sudden onset of right flank pain which radiates to the groin. She explains that the pain comes in waves and is associated with nausea. On examination she is writhing about in pain, she has a temperature of 36.6°C, heart rate of 94 beats per minute and a BP of 110/88 mmHg. She is tender in the right flank. Urine dipstick reveals haematuria.

5. A 21-year-old woman presents with a two-day history of pelvic pain and dyspareunia. She also reports offensive vaginal discharge. On examination, chandelier sign is positive. She has been with her current sexual partner for the past two months.

See pages 144–145 for answers.

ANSWERS

Amenorrhoea 1

1. **K. Turner syndrome**
   This is a condition that results from a complete deletion of all or part of the X chromosome. Patients with this condition present with primary amenorrhoea, they also have poorly developed or absent secondary sexual characteristics.

2. **I. Primary ovarian insufficiency**
   This is a condition in which the ovaries fail to function effectively before the age of 40.

3. **H. Pregnancy**
   This should be considered in every sexually active woman of childbearing age who presents with secondary amenorrhoea. It is believed that the vomiting in pregnancy is directly linked to the rising HCG levels.

4. **G. Polycystic ovarian syndrome**
   This patient has signs of hyperandrogenism and menstrual irregularities. She meets two out of three criteria for PCOS as per the Rotterdam criteria.

5. **J. Prolactinoma**
   This is a non-cancerous tumor of the pituitary gland which causes an elevation in prolactin. Clinical features can include visual changes due to compression on the optic chiasm, headaches, galactorrhoea and amenorrhoea.

6. **D. Hypothyroidism**
   This patient presents with amenorrhoea, weight gain, constipation, cold intolerance, dry skin and hair thinning. All of these symptoms are associated with hypothyroidism.

Amenorrhoea 2

1. **B. Congenital adrenal hyperplasia**
   CAH is an inherited group of conditions which affect the adrenal glands. Classical laboratory findings include hypoglycaemia, hyponatraemia, hyperkalaemia and an elevated 17α-hydroxyprogesterone level.

2. **E. Kallmann syndrome**
   This condition is a form of hypogonadotropic hypogonadism and is characterised by delayed or absent puberty. Patients also typically have a history of anosmia.

3. **A. Anorexia nervosa**
   Amenorrhoea in anorexia nervosa is related to hypothalamic dysfunction.

4. **C. Cushing syndrome**
   This condition results from an excessive amount of the hormone cortisol in the body. It can result in amenorrhoea, hypertension, moon facies, abdominal striae and muscle wasting as seen in this patient.

5. **F. Menopause**
   This is a point in a woman's life where she ceases to have periods. This patient also has hot flushes and night sweats which are common symptoms of menopause.

Breast pathology 1

1. J. Mastitis
This is inflammation of the breast tissue and is common amongst breast feeding women.

2. K. Mondor disease
This results from thrombophlebitis of a superficial vein of the breast.

3. I. Lactating adenoma
These are well circumscribed masses that commonly develop during the last trimester of pregnancy or shortly after pregnancy.

4. G. Fibroadenoma
These are common benign breast lesions. Pushing on a fibroadenoma can cause it to move away from beneath your fingers, for this reason some people refer to them as breast mice.

5. P. Phyllodes tumor
These present as painless mobile breast lumps which grow fairly rapidly. They can cause ulceration of the skin overlying the lump.

Breast pathology 2

1. E. Ductal ectasia
This is a benign condition that results from widening and thickening of milk ducts within the breast. Patients (if symptomatic) typically present complaining of green-brown coloured discharge, nipple inversion or a palpable lump.

2. F. Fat necrosis
Fat necrosis in the breast is a lump of dead tissue that typically results from trauma to the affected breast.

3. L. Nipple thrush
This patient presents with persistent nipple pain after a course of antibiotics

4. C. Breast lymphoma
This patient presents with clinical features and medical history suggestive of breast implant related lymphoma.

5. B. Breast cyst
This patient presents with a breast lump and ultrasound findings consistent with a cyst. Needle aspiration shows a clear fluid from within the lesion and aspiration causes resolution of the mass.

6. D. Ductal carcinoma in situ
DCIS usually presents without symptoms. Mammography reveals tiny specks of calcium called calcifications; diagnosis is confirmed by biopsy.

Breast pathology 3

1. A. Breast abscess
If mastitis due to breast feeding is not treated promptly a breast abscess can form.

2. N. Paget's disease of the breast
This is a condition that occurs mostly in women over the age of 50. The most common symptom is an eczema like rash over the nipple.

3. H. Galactocele

These are milk filled cysts that are caused by lactiferous duct occlusion. They are typically found in breast feeding mothers.

4. M. Nipple vasospasm

Also known as Raynaud's phenomenon of the nipple, it is caused by tightening and vasospasm of blood vessels and can result in white discoloration of the nipple.

5. O. Papilloma

This patient has unilateral bloody discharge from her left breast and there is no palpable lump on examination.

Menstrual irregularities 1

1. B. Cervical ectropion

Patients are mostly asymptomatic but can have light bleeding post-sexual intercourse or intermenstrual bleeds. Speculum examination reveals a bright red and rough cervix. The visible changes are as a result of glandular cells which line the cervical canal extending to the outer surface of the cervix.

2. H. Polycystic ovarian syndrome

This is a condition in which there are signs and symptoms of excessive androgens. This patient has irregular periods, physical findings of hyperandrogenism and ultrasound findings suggestive of PCOS.

3. I. Uterine Fibroid

Also known as leiomyomas, this patient has a typical ultrasound finding. They are a common cause of menorrhagia.

4. D. Endometrial cancer

Postmenopausal vaginal bleeding should be considered as cancer until proven otherwise.

5. E. Endometriosis

This occurs when tissue similar to that which lines the uterus is found growing outside of the uterus. Patients typically complain of pain with menses. Diagnosis is confirmed with laparoscopy.

6. K. Von Willebrand disease

This patient has a history of heavy menstrual bleeds and family history of prolonged bleeds. Her symptoms are worsened by the use of an NSAID. Her blood results and history indicate a diagnosis of Von Willebrand disease.

Menstrual irregularities 2

1. J. Uterine polyp

This patient has the characteristic "interrupted mucosa sign" on ultrasound examination.

2. F. Factor X deficiency

This is a condition in which coagulation takes a longer period of time than normal. In women this can cause prolonged and heavy menstrual cycles.

3. A. Adenomyosis

This occurs when the endometrial tissue which normally lines the uterus starts to grow into the muscle layer of the uterus.

4. C. Dysfunctional uterine bleeding

This is any vaginal bleeding that varies from the normal menstrual cycle of a woman that is not due to pregnancy, pelvic or systemic infection.

5. G. Hypothyroidism

This patient has symptoms and physical signs suggestive of hypothyroidism as a cause for her presentation with menorrhagia.

Male infertility 1

1. H. Varicocele

This is an enlargement of veins within the scrotum. Varicoceles are commonly associated with decreased sperm production and infertility.

2. C. Del Castillo syndrome

In this condition only Sertoli cells line the seminiferous tubules where sperm normally develop, this results in absence of sperm in the tubules.

3. F. Klinefelter syndrome

This is a genetic condition which affects males. This condition can cause infertility as most males with this condition cannot produce enough sperm. The testes are commonly affected and are smaller than normal.

4. E. Kallmann syndrome

This condition is a form of hypogonadotropic hypogonadism and is characterised by delayed or absent puberty. Patients also typically have a history of anosmia.

Male infertility 2

1. G. Primary ciliary dyskinesia

This is a genetic condition which affects cilia within the airways and can cause recurrent respiratory tract infections. Patients are also at an increased risk of bronchiectasis. Patients with this condition can present with situs inversus and dextrocardia.

2. A. Cryptorchidism

Testicles are normally palpable within the scrotum, occasionally during development one or even both of the testicles may not descend into the scrotum. In adult males this may cause infertility.

3. I. Young's syndrome

This condition results in infertility due to obstruction of the vas deferens and is commonly associated with chronic rhinosinusitis.

4. B. Drug induced infertility

Anabolic steroids can interfere with the hormonal systems that are involved with sperm production thus resulting in infertility.

5. D. Hyperprolactinaemia

This results from a non-cancerous tumor of the pituitary gland which causes an elevation in prolactin. Clinical features can include visual changes due to compression on the optic chiasm and headaches. In females galactorrhoea and amenorrhoea can also occur.

Complications of pregnancy 1

1. G. Missed miscarriage

This is where the fetus has died but remains in the uterus. Ultrasound is the best way of confirming diagnosis.

2. A. Blighted ovum

This is a form of pregnancy in which the embryo does not develop.

3. E. Hydatidiform mole

These occur when the placenta grows irregularly and rapidly. Sacs of fluid develop within the placenta and can resemble a bunch of grapes on ultrasound examination. In these pregnancies patients have all of the common symptoms of pregnancy as the placenta produces hCG.

4. B. Chorioamnionitis

This is a maternal infection that results from migration of bacteria from the vagina into the uterus. This patient has presented beyond 20 weeks of gestation with a fever, lower abdominal pain, tachycardia and foul-smelling discharge.

5. I. Threatened miscarriage

This is defined as vaginal bleeding before 20 weeks completed gestation with a closed cervix.

Complications of pregnancy 2

1. F. Inevitable miscarriage

This patient has heavy bleeding, abdominal pain and an open cervix.

2. C. Complete miscarriage

This occurs when all of the products of conception have left the uterus.

3. D. Cornual pregnancy

This is a rare form of ectopic pregnancy in which the fertilised egg implants itself in one of the horns of the uterus.

4. H. Recurrent miscarriage.

This is defined as three or more consecutive pregnancy losses.

Vulvovaginal pathology 1

1. G. Lichen sclerosus

This condition affects postmenopausal women more often and presents as thinned skin in the vulva which is patchy in appearance.

2. J. Psoriasis

Genital psoriasis is a common condition, diagnosis is made based on clinical findings and history.

3. C. Bartholin's cyst

Bartholin's glands are pea sized structures found on each side of the vaginal opening and secrete fluids that help lubricate the vagina. If these glands become blocked a cyst can form which is usually unilateral.

4. A. Allergic contact dermatitis

The lesions described are typical of this and the history of using a new feminine hygiene product are consistent with this.

Vulvovaginal pathology 2

1. D. Condyloma acuminata

Otherwise known as genital warts, this condition is commonly spread from skin to skin contact during sexual intercourse. A virus called human papillomavirus causes the warts to develop.

2. B. Atrophic vaginitis

Atrophic vaginitis in this context is likely associated with the decreased level of estrogen that occurs during lactation.

3. L. Vulvovaginal candidiasis

This is a condition in which there is overgrowth of yeast within the vagina. Women present with symptoms including itch, burning sensations and vaginal discharge.

4. E. Folliculitis

This patient has presented with hot tub folliculitis which is due to infection of the skin. This condition is most commonly caused by *Pseudomonas aeruginosa*.

5. I. Molluscum contagiosum

This is an infection caused by the pox virus. Lesions are typically described as clusters of umbilicated papules.

Female infertility 1

1. G. Hypogonadotrophic hypogonadism

GnRH is normally released by the hypothalamus, this results in FSH and LH release from the pituitary gland. These two hormones in women are involved with folliculogenesis. In hypogonadotrophic hypogonadism there is reduced GnRH release and this results in reduction of LH and FSH, causing infertility.

2. B. Cushing syndrome

In this condition there is an elevated level of cortisol, this can cause cessation or irregularity of the menstrual cycle. This can cause difficulties with fertility.

3. J. Uterine fibroid

These can cause infertility by distortion of normal anatomy of the cervix and uterus, limiting the entry of sperm, obstructing the fallopian tubes and limiting uterine blood flow thereby reducing the ability for embryo implantation.

4. I. Premature ovarian failure

This condition occurs when the ovaries stop their normal function prior to the age of 40. Diagnosis requires FSH elevation greater than 40 on two separate occasions at least four to six weeks apart and at least six months of amenorrhoea.

Female infertility 2

1. E. Hashimoto's thyroiditis

Most individuals with this condition develop hypothyroidism. Low levels of thyroid hormones can impair ovulation thus leading to difficulties with conception.

2. H. Polycystic ovarian syndrome

This is a condition in which patients present with two of three features as outlined by the Rotterdam criteria. This patient presents with two of these:

menstrual irregularities and hyperandrogenism. The third criterion is polycystic ovaries visualised on ultrasound examination.

3. A. Asherman's syndrome

This is an acquired condition in which scar tissue forms within the uterus or around the cervix. The scar tissue causes the uterus walls to adhere to one another.

4. C. Endometriosis

This occurs when tissue similar to that which lines the uterus is found growing outside of the uterus. Patients typically complain of pain with menses. Diagnosis is confirmed with laparoscopy. Infertility is a common complication of endometriosis.

5. F. Hyperprolactinaemia

This condition is as a result of excessive prolactin production. Elevated prolactin decreases estrogen production and impairs ovulation, this can lead to infertility.

Obstetric complications 1

1. I. Preterm premature rupture of membranes

This is defined as rupture of membranes prior to 37 weeks' gestation. Fluid within the vagina should raise suspicion of PPROM. Diagnosis is achieved by maternal history and sterile speculum exam. Nitrazine paper turns blue in the presence of amniotic fluid as a result of pH > 6. The fern test can also be performed, this involves taking a swab of the vaginal fluid and placing it on a glass slide, you expect to observe ferning of the dried fluid on microscopy.

2. B. Eclampsia

This patient has presented with eclampsia, she has a persistently elevated blood pressure, neurological symptoms (headache), proteinuria and is having a seizure. She requires urgent review and management for her presentation.

3. H. Pre-Eclampsia

This patient has presented with pre-eclampsia, she has a persistently elevated blood pressure, neurological symptoms (headache) and proteinuria. She requires prompt review and management for her presentation.

4. E. Placental abruption

This patient has presented with sudden onset abdominal pain, continuous contractions, vaginal bleeding and fetal distress.

5. A. Amniotic fluid embolism

This is a life-threatening complication of childbirth in which amniotic fluid enters the blood stream. The resulting reaction can cause coagulopathy, heart and lung failure.

Obstetric complications 2

1. K. Shoulder dystocia

This is an obstetric emergency in which the head is delivered and the anterior shoulder is caught in the mother's pubic bone. The head characteristically retracts (Turtle sign).

2. C. Ectopic pregnancy

This patient presents with a positive urine HCG and an empty uterus. She also has severe abdominal pain and evidence of internal bleeding (hypotension and tachycardia).

3. G. Postpartum haemorrhage

This is a serious, life-threatening complication of child birth. This patient has presented with evidence of an atonic uterus, a major contributing factor to postpartum haemorrhage.

4. F. Placenta praevia

This is where the placenta implants itself at the base of the uterus above the cervix, preventing vaginal delivery. Patients typically present with painless vaginal bleeding in the third trimester.

5. J. Prolapsed umbilical cord

When the cord is prolapsed, it may be squeezed between the baby and the womb during contractions, this reduces oxygen supply to the fetus and is an obstetric emergency. The heart rate of child will typically slow after the waters break.

Dysmenorrhoea

1. F. Fibroid

Also known as leiomyomas this patient has a typical ultrasound findings of a uterine fibroid. They are a common cause of menorrhagia.

2. E. Endometriosis

This occurs when tissue similar to that which lines the uterus is found growing outside of the uterus. Patients typically complain of pain with menses. Diagnosis is confirmed with laparoscopy.

3. C. Cervical stenosis

This is a possible complication of LLETZ procedure.

4. J. Pelvic inflammatory disease

This occurs when a vaginal infection passes to the cervix, the uterus and fallopian tubes. The most common causes of this presentation are chlamydia and gonorrhoea.

6. D. Ectopic pregnancy

This patient presents with a positive urine HCG and an empty uterus. She also has severe abdominal pain and vaginal bleeding.

Sexually Transmitted Infection 1

1. C. Chlamydia trachomatis

This is a common sexually transmitted infection which in women can cause damage to the reproductive system and cause difficulties with fertility.

2. A. Bacterial vaginosis

This condition results in inflammatory changes of the vagina as a result of overgrowth of bacteria, which is normally found within the vagina. Typical features include vaginal irritation, dysuria and foul-smelling discharge.

3. G. Human papillomavirus

This is a very common sexually transmitted infection which can be asymptomatic. Human papillomavirus results in genital warts and can cause cervical cancer.

4. E. Genital herpes

This is a sexually transmitted infection which results in painful vesicular lesions. It is caused by the herpes simplex virus.

Sexually Transmitted Infection 2

1. J. Trichomoniasis

This is a common sexually transmitted infection caused by *Trichomonas vaginalis*, a protozoan parasite. This patient presents with vaginal itch and discharge. Speculum examination reveals a strawberry cervix which is a sign that is very common with this infection.

2. F. Gonorrhoea

This is a sexually transmitted infection caused by the bacterium *Neisseria gonorrhoea*. This patient has presented with classic symptoms of gonorrhoea infection including penile discharge, dysuria and testicular pain.

3. B. Candidiasis

This is a condition in which there is overgrowth of yeast within the vagina. Women present with symptoms including itch, burning sensations and vaginal discharge which is typically described as being of a cottage cheese appearance.

4. I. Syphilis

This is a sexually transmitted infection caused by a bacteria called *Treponema pallidum*. This patient has presented with symptoms consistent with syphilis, including primary chancre on his penis and lymph node enlargement.

Genetic disorders 1

1. F. Marfan syndrome

This condition is inherited as an autosomal dominant trait.

2. B. Down syndrome (Trisomy 21)

This is a genetic condition in which a child is born with an additional copy of chromosome 21.

3. J. Williams syndrome

This is a genetic condition caused by deletion of genes on chromosome 7.

4. D. Fragile X syndrome

This is a genetic condition caused by a change to one of the genes on the X chromosome. Patients with this condition typically present with intellectual disabilities.

Genetic disorders 2

1. G. Noonan syndrome

This is a genetic condition caused by mutation in the PTPN11 gene on chromosome 12.

2. E. Klinefelter syndrome (XXY)

This is a genetic condition in which males are born with an additional copy of the X chromosome.

3. I. Turner's syndrome

This is a genetic condition in females in which an X chromosome is completely or partially absent.

4. A. Angelman syndrome

This is a genetic condition caused by a defect with chromosome 15.

Pelvic-Abdominal pain 1

1. K. Ruptured ectopic pregnancy

This patient presents with a positive urine HCG and an empty uterus. She also has severe abdominal pain and evidence of internal bleeding (hypotension and tachycardia).

2. E. Mittelschmerz

Also known as ovulation pain this occurs midway through a woman's menstrual cycle.

3. L. Ruptured ovarian cyst

These are a common cause of acute pelvic pain in pre-menopausal women. Cysts usually do not cause patients to become symptomatic but can rupture after strenuous physical activity or sexual intercourse.

4. A. Appendicitis

The pain of appendicitis commences around the umbilicus and eventually radiates to the right iliac fossa as a result of peritoneal irritation.

5. D. Endometritis

This condition results from inflammation of the lining of the uterus. This condition can be associated with retained products of conception after surgical termination of pregnancy.

Pelvic-Abdominal pain 2

1. F. Ovarian hyperstimulation syndrome

This is a complication of assisted reproduction treatment. As a result of hormone therapy, the ovaries swell and become painful.

2. C. Endometriosis

In this condition the tissue which normally lines the uterus, known as the endometrium, grows outside of the uterus. This can cause significantly painful menstrual cycles as a result of peritoneal irritation. Endometrial nodules in the pouch of Douglas are a common finding.

3. G. Ovarian torsion

Common ultrasound findings are ovarian swelling, decreased or absent venous flow, free pelvic fluid and there may be a positive follicular ring sign.

4. J. Renal calculus

Renal calculi are hard deposits that form within the kidney. Passage of stones can be quite painful; the pain is usually described as being in loin to groin distribution.

5. H. Pelvic inflammatory disease

This occurs when a vaginal infection passes to the cervix, the uterus and fallopian tubes. The most common causes of this presentation are chlamydia and gonorrhoea.

Urology

6

PENIS DISORDERS

A. Balanitis xerotica obliterans
B. Epispadias
C. Hirsutoid papillomas
D. Hypospadias
E. Lichen planus
F. Paraphimosis
G. Penile fracture
H. Penile Mondor's disease
 I. Penile wart
J. Peyronie's disease
K. Phimosis
L. Priapism

For each of the following, what is the MOST likely diagnosis?

1. A 37-year-old male presents to your emergency department with acute onset severe pain in his penis for the past two hours. During a particularly rough episode of coitus his penis withdrew and on trying to attempt vaginal penetration he heard a cracking sound as his partner pushed up against it, this was followed by detumescence.
2. A 3-year-old boy is brought into your emergency department with painful swelling in his glans for the past six hours. His mother tells you that she has been unable to protract his foreskin after he pulled it back while playing in the bath at home. On examination the glans is congested and enlarged with a collar of swollen foreskin at the base of the glans.
3. A 3-year-old is brought by his mother. She is concerned as she has not been able to retract his foreskin while showering him. When he urinates, she has noticed ballooning of his foreskin.
4. A mother brings in a 6-month-old who has been urinating irregularly. There seems to be urine exiting from the underside of his penis. On examination you note an opening in the ventral surface of the penis between the glans and the scrotum.
5. A woman has just given birth to a male child who you are asked to review. On examination you find an opening in the ventral surface of the penis, shortly

DOI: 10.1201/9781003459941-6

after observing this the child begins to passage urine through it. The remainder of the examination is unremarkable.

6. A 21-year-old man presents with a one-week history of dorsal induration. He reports that he has had a constant ache and throbbing sensation in the penis for the duration. He has no systemic symptoms and reports he has been otherwise well. On examination there is a rope like cord which is palpable on the dorsum of the penis proximally.

7. A 36-year-old uncircumcised male presents to your clinic complaining of difficulty urinating. He reports that his stream is crooked and he has also noted changes on his penis. On examination the glans of the penis appears white in color, firm and scarred, particularly around the meatus which appears stenosed.

See page 154 for answers.

TESTICULAR AND SCROTAL DISORDERS 1

A. Alcock canal syndrome
B. Angiokeratoma of Fordyce
C. Candidal intertrigo
D. Fournier's gangrene
E. Gumma of the testis
F. Henoch–Schönlein purpura
G. Hydrocele
H. Epididymo-Orchitis
I. Male genital dysaesthesia
J. Retractile testicle
K. Scrotal abscess
L. Scrotal calcinosis
M. Seminoma
N. Sperm granuloma
O. Spermatocele
P. Teratoma
Q. Testicular torsion
R. Tinea cruris
S. Torsion of hydatid of Morgagni
T. Undescended testicle
U. Varicocele

For each of the following, what is the MOST likely diagnosis?

1. A 6-year-old boy presents to your emergency department with acute swelling and pain in the left hemi-scrotum associated with macroscopic haematuria. On examination there is scrotal swelling and the testicles are easily palpable, non-tender and of normal size. You note that he has a non-blanching rash over his left scrotum, buttocks and extensor surfaces of the lower limbs.

2. A 42-year-old man presents to your GP clinic concerned about a lump above his left testicle. He has no recent illness and has no significant medical history. On examination there is a non-tender fluctuant swelling in the upper part of the posterior left testicle. The right and left testes are easily palpable.

3. A 28-year-old male presents to your clinic complaining of a two-day history of scrotal pain and swelling. On examination he has a temperature of 38.1°C and there is an erythematous, tender, fluctuant mass measuring 3 cm on the right hemi-scrotum.

4. A mother brings a 3-month-old infant to your clinic. She is concerned as she could not palpate his testicles when she was changing his nappy the day prior to attendance. On examination you palpate a single testicle in the scrotum, you are able to coax the second testicle into the scrotum with gentle palpation.

5. A 26-year-old male presents with a painless swollen right testicle. He explains that it has progressively enlarged over the past month and he is concerned. On examination there is fluctuation, the testicle is not palpable and there is positive transillumination.

6. A 13-year-old male presents to your emergency department with severe pain in his right scrotum which radiates to right lower quadrant abdomen. His symptoms started suddenly 45 minutes prior; he has vomited twice in your assessment bay. His mother reports that he was born with a bell clapper deformity affecting both testicles. On examination Prehn's sign is negative and the cremasteric reflex is absent.

See pages 154–155 for answers.

TESTICULAR AND SCROTAL DISORDERS 2

A. Alcock canal syndrome
B. Angiokeratoma of Fordyce
C. Candidal intertrigo
D. Fournier's gangrene
E. Gumma of the testis
F. Henoch–Schönlein purpura
G. Hydrocele
H. Epididymo-Orchitis
I. Male genital dysaesthesia

J. **Retractile testicle**
K. **Scrotal abscess**
L. **Scrotal calcinosis**
M. **Seminoma**
N. **Sperm granuloma**
O. **Spermatocele**
P. **Teratoma**
Q. **Testicular torsion**
R. **Tinea cruris**
S. **Torsion of hydatid of Morgagni**
T. **Undescended testicle**
U. **Varicocele**

For each of the following, what is the MOST likely diagnosis?

1. A 42-year-old man presents with a two-week history of swelling and pain in the left testicle. The pain commenced five days ago. On questioning he reports that he has had multiple male partners over the past 12 months. Examination reveals a left testicle which has a "billiard ball" like hard consistency and inguinal lymph node enlargement in bilateral groins. An EIA is initially requested and this returns reactive, a diagnosis is subsequently confirmed with a positive RPR.

2. A 39-year-old male presents to your clinic complaining of non-painful nodules in the left side of his scrotum. The lumps started as small nodules but have progressively enlarged over the past eight months. He has no history of trauma and has been with the same sexual partner for five years. On examination he has a temperature of 36.7°C, you observe two nodules in the left hemi-scrotum which are yellow in color and measure 0.3 cm and 0.2 cm. The nodules are hard, firm and there is no surrounding erythema.

3. A 10-year-old boy presents with a 12-hour history of pain in the left testicle. He has no history of trauma or recent illness. On examination there is a blue tender lump at the upper pole of the left testicle.

4. A 27-year-old male presents to your clinic with a three-month history of rash on his left hemi-scrotum and groin which is very itchy. It started off as a small area but has progressively increased. On examination there is a well demarcated scaly plaque with raised borders and central clearing which extends from the left groin into the scrotum.

5. A 38-year-old male presents to your clinic concerned about a lump he has noticed in his right testicle. He has had a loss of appetite and has lost 5 kg in the past three months. He had an undescended testicle as a child and had surgery to correct this, otherwise he has no significant medical history. On examination you can palpate a hard painless lump in the right testicle. You arrange for laboratory investigations which reveal a normal AFP and a slightly elevated HCG.

See page 155 for answers.

TESTICULAR AND SCROTAL DISORDERS 3

A. Alcock canal syndrome
B. Angiokeratoma of Fordyce
C. Candidal intertrigo
D. Fournier's gangrene
E. Gumma of the testis
F. Henoch–Schönlein purpura
G. Hydrocele
H. Epididymo-Orchitis
I. Male genital dysaesthesia
J. Retractile testicle
K. Scrotal abscess
L. Scrotal calcinosis
M. Seminoma
N. Sperm granuloma
O. Spermatocele
P. Teratoma
Q. Testicular torsion
R. Tinea cruris
S. Torsion of hydatid of Morgagni
T. Undescended testicle
U. Varicocele

For each of the following, what is the MOST likely diagnosis?

1. A 54-year-old obese, diabetic male presents to your clinic complaining of a four-week history of itch in his right groin extending onto his scrotum. On examination there are multiple erythematous and macerated plaques in the right groin extending to the right hemi-scrotum. You also note peripheral scaling and satellite papules.

2. A 39-year-old man presents with swelling in his left hemi-scrotum. On examination there is swelling on the left side which on palpation feels like a "bag of worms"; the swelling decreases in size when he is supine.

3. A 37-year-old male attends your clinic as he is concerned about some spots which he has noticed on his scrotum which are bumpy and rough to touch. On examination of his scrotum, you note three dark purple papules, measuring 3 mm at most, with a rough surface.

4. A 65-year-old obese, type 2 diabetic presents to your emergency department complaining of a three-hour history of severe pain in the left hemi-scrotum. On examination he has a temperature of 38.6°C and you note an area of dark red skin measuring 2 cm in diameter in the left hemi-scrotum. The area of concern

is extremely tender to palpation and the tenderness extends beyond the border of the demarcated erythema; you also note crepitus.

5. A 21-year-old male presents with a left sided testicular lump. He noticed it yesterday while showering and reports that he is otherwise well. He is concerned as his father had testicular cancer. He had an undescended testicle as a child. On examination you note an irregular hard painless lump in the left testicle. You arrange for laboratory investigations which reveal elevated AFP and HCG.

6. A 35-year-old competitive long-distance cyclist presents to your clinic complaining of recurrent and prolonged pain in the penis and scrotum while sitting down. He reports that his symptoms are relieved by standing. He also reports that he has been experiencing similar pain during intercourse.

See pages 155–156 for answers.

UROLOGY 1

A. **Acute interstitial nephritis**
B. **Acute post-streptococcal glomerulonephritis**
C. **Acute prostatitis**
D. **Acute tubular necrosis**
E. **Benign prostatic hyperplasia**
F. **Chronic prostatitis**
G. **Cystitis**
H. **IgA nephropathy**
I. **Polycystic kidney disease**
J. **Prostate cancer**
K. **Pyelonephritis**
L. **Renal calculus**
M. **Renal cell carcinoma**
N. **Wilms tumor**

For each of the following, what is the MOST likely diagnosis?

1. A 39-year-old man presents with worsening right flank pain for the past three months. He explains that he also suffers from night sweats and has lost 8 kg during this time. He has no significant medical history and is not using any medication. On examination he has a palpable mass in the right flank. Urine dipstick reveals microscopic haematuria.

2. A 67-year-old male attends your clinic complaining of a three-month history of difficulty with initiation of micturition, when it does get started, he reports dribbling and a feeling of incomplete emptying of the bladder. He noticed some blood in his urine the other day. He denies any associated pain and has no loss of appetite or weight.

3. A 29-year-old man attended his regular GP yesterday with reduced urine output. His GP arranged for some blood tests which revealed an acute drop in his eGFR and an elevated creatinine. His blood tests two weeks ago were normal while in hospital for abdominal pain. While in hospital he was given plenty of analgesia and commenced on IV gentamicin which was continued until his discharge one week later. On examination he has pitting edema in bilateral lower limbs. You observe that there are muddy brown casts on urinalysis.

4. A 66-year-old female presents with a two-day history of haematuria, dysuria, frequency and foul-smelling urine. On examination she has a temperature of 37.1°C and she has tenderness in the suprapubic region of her abdomen.

5. An 11-year-old boy presents to your emergency department with his mother who is concerned about swelling of his face. He has no significant past medical history and last attended his GP nine days ago for treatment of tonsillitis. On examination his vitals are normal. There is edema of the lower limbs up to his shins bilaterally, also in the scrotum and face. Dipstick of his urine reveals haematuria and proteinuria. Antistreptolysine O antibody levels are elevated.

See page 156 for answers.

UROLOGY 2

A. **Acute interstitial nephritis**
B. **Acute post-streptococcal glomerulonephritis**
C. **Acute prostatitis**
D. **Acute tubular necrosis**
E. **Benign prostatic hyperplasia**
F. **Chronic prostatitis**
G. **Cystitis**
H. **IgA nephropathy**
I. **Polycystic kidney disease**
J. **Prostate cancer**
K. **Pyelonephritis**
L. **Renal calculus**
M. **Renal cell carcinoma**
N. **Wilms tumor**

For each of the following, what is the MOST likely diagnosis?

1. A 65-year-old male presents to your clinic complaining of a four-month history of fatigue and lower back pain which wakes him at night. He reports that he has woken up in the middle of the night on several occasions with the urge to

urinate. His stream is weak and he has terminal dribbling. He reports that he has lost 3 kg during this time.

2. A 25-year-old woman presents to your clinic complaining of fever, body aches and dark colored urine. She has recently had mastitis and has been commenced on cephalexin for treatment of this. On examination she has a temperature of 38.4°C, blood pressure of 136/94 mmHg and there is a maculopapular rash across her body. Urinalysis is performed and reveals proteinuria, eosinophilia, five to ten red blood cells per hpf and five to ten white blood cells per hpf.

3. A 3-year-old boy is brought by his mother who noticed that he appeared swollen over the left flank, he has been well otherwise and has not complained of any pain or discomfort. On examination there is a palpable left flank mass which is non tender. Urine dipstick reveals haematuria.

4. A 29-year-old man presents with a six-hour history of frank haematuria, colicky right groin and abdominal pain. He has also vomited multiple times. On examination he is writhing about in pain, he has a temperature of 36.3°C, heart rate of 88 beats per minute and a BP of 116/82 mmHg. He is tender in the right flank. Urine dipstick reveals haematuria.

5. A 45-year-old male presents with a four-month history of fatigue associated with perineal and rectal pain. He also reports that he has been experiencing dysuria. Examination of the abdomen and flanks is unremarkable, rectal exam reveals a tender prostate gland. A two-glass test is performed which reveals > 20 leukocytes per hpf on the post massage urine sample.

See page 157 for answers.

ANSWERS

Penis disorders

1. G. Penile fracture

The correct answer is Penile fracture. This condition occurs as a result of a tear in the tunica albuginea, a tough fibrous layer of tissue which surrounds the corpora cavernosa.

2. F. Paraphimosis

The correct answer is paraphimosis. This is a condition in which the foreskin becomes trapped around the glans of the uncircumcised penis. This is a medical emergency and requires urgent reduction.

3. K. Phimosis

The correct answer is phimosis. This is a common condition seen in uncircumcised children and typically resolves by the age of seven. Ballooning or bulging of the foreskin during micturition may warrant urological review.

4. D. Hypospadias

The correct answer is hypospadias. This is a condition in which the opening of the urethra is located on the underside of the penis or scrotum rather than at the tip of the penis.

5. B. Epispadias

The correct answer is epispadias. This is a condition in which the opening of the urethra is located on the dorsum of the penis rather than at the tip of the penis.

6. H. Penile Mondor's disease

The correct answer is penile Mondor's disease. This condition, also known as penile dorsal vein thrombosis, results in thrombophlebitis in the superficial dorsal vein of the penis.

7. A. Balanitis xerotica obliterans

The correct answer is balanitis xerotica obliterans. Also known as penile lichen sclerosus, this condition usually affects the glans and the foreskin. Patients complain of urinary stream difficulties, painful erections and difficulty retracting their foreskins.

Testicular and scrotal disorders 1

1. G. Henoch–Schönlein purpura

The correct answer is Henoch–Schönlein purpura. This is a condition in which small blood vessels become inflamed and bleed. Patients typically present with a characteristic purple rash in the lower limbs and buttocks, they also report abdominal pain and joint pain. The scrotum can be involved and must be distinguished from testicular torsion.

2. O. Spermatocele

The correct answer is spermatocele. Also known as an epididymal cyst, this is a painless fluid filled cyst which forms in the epididymis, a structure which lies above and behind each testicle.

3. K. Scrotal abscess

The correct answer is scrotal abscess. Examination typically reveals an oedematous and erythematous scrotum with a fluctuant mass. There are many causes behind scrotal abscess formation.

4. J. Retractile testicle

The correct answer is retractile testicle. This is a testicle that moves between the scrotum and the groin. Unlike an undescended testicle it can be guided back into the scrotum during physical exam.

5. H. Hydrocele

The correct answer is hydrocele. This is an accumulation of fluid between the parietal and visceral layers of the tunica vaginalis. It usually presents as painless swelling in the scrotum.

6. Q. Testicular torsion

The correct answer is testicular torsion. This is a medical emergency which requires urgent treatment to save the affected testicle. This condition results from rotation and twisting of the spermatic cord; this causes the blood flow to the affected testicle to be cut off. A bell clapper testicle is a risk factor for testicular torsion.

Testicular and scrotal disorders 2

1. F. Gumma of the testis

The correct answer is gumma of the testis. The syphilitic testicular gumma classically presents as a "billiard ball" like testicle, which is firm, hard and round. The gumma may be hard to distinguish from a tumor on examination.

2. L. Scrotal calcinosis

The correct answer is scrotal calcinosis. This is a benign condition which is characterised by the presence of a solitary or multiple calcified nodules in the scrotal skin.

3. S. Torsion of hydatid of Morgagni

The correct answer is torsion of hydatid of Morgagni. This patient has the classic blue dot sign which represents an ischaemic appendix testicle.

4. R. Tinea cruris

The correct answer is tinea cruris. Also known as jock itch, this is a fungal infection which causes a red itchy rash in warm and moist areas such as the groin.

5. M. Seminoma

The correct answer is seminoma. This type of testicular cancer mostly affects men between the ages of 30 and 40 whereas teratoma usually affects younger males.

Testicular and scrotal disorders 3

1. C. Candidal intertrigo

The correct answer is candidal intertrigo. This is a skin infection caused by growth of candida species. This patient has risk factors for development of this condition including obesity and diabetes mellitus.

2. U. Varicocele

The correct answer is varicocele. This presentation occurs as a result of dilatation of the pampiniform plexus of veins within the spermatic cord. They are typically described as a "bag of worms", most commonly occur on the left side and are reduced in size when supine as gravity no longer fills the plexus.

3. B. Angiokeratoma of Fordyce

The correct answer is angiokeratoma of Fordyce. These are asymptomatic benign skin lesions. Histologically they are thin-walled vessels in the superficial dermis of the skin with overlying hyperplasia.

4. E. Fournier's gangrene

The correct answer is Fournier's gangrene. This is a form of necrotizing fasciitis which commonly affects the genitalia and is more commonly found in diabetics.

5. P. Teratoma

The correct answer is teratoma. This type of testicular cancer mostly affects younger men between the ages of 20 and 30 whereas seminoma usually affects older males. Seminomas by definition do not secrete AFP.

6. A. Alcock canal syndrome

The correct answer is Alcock canal syndrome. Also known as pudendal nerve entrapment syndrome or cyclist syndrome, this condition is caused by compression of the pudendal nerve. Patients complain of pain or insensitivity in perineal sites. Symptoms can be exacerbated by sitting and are usually relieved by standing.

Urology 1

1. M. Renal cell carcinoma

The correct answer is renal cell carcinoma. This patient has the classic triad of features including; haematuria, flank pain and a palpable flank mass. This patient also presents with constitutional features: weight loss and night sweats.

2. E. Prostatic hyperplasia

The correct answer is prostatic hyperplasia. This is a common condition which results in lower urinary tract symptoms secondary to prostate enlargement.

3. D. Acute tubular necrosis

The correct answer is acute tubular necrosis. This condition results from the destruction of the tubular epithelial cells which make up the renal tubules of the kidneys. Patients present with acute kidney injury. In this case the most likely cause of the injury is the use of gentamicin. The presence of muddy brown casts on urinalysis is pathognomonic for acute tubular necrosis.

4. G. Cystitis

The correct answer is cystitis. This is an infection of the bladder which almost always has a bacterial cause. This patient has classical features of this.

5. B. Acute post-streptococcal glomerulonephritis

The correct answer is acute post-streptococcal glomerulonephritis. This is a condition of the kidney which can develop after a group A streptococcal infection. This commonly presents with features of nephritic syndrome one to two weeks after streptococcal throat infections.

Urology 2

1. **J. Prostate cancer**

   The correct answer is prostate cancer. This patient has features of metastatic prostate carcinoma including chronic lower back pain associated with loss of weight and symptoms of prostatism.

2. **A. Acute interstitial nephritis**

   The correct answer is acute interstitial nephritis. This patient has presented with classic features of this condition: a fever, generalised maculopapular rash, haematuria and eosinophiluria. This presentation is a result of cephalosporin use.

3. **N. Wilms tumor**

   The correct answer is Wilms tumor. Also known as a nephroblastoma, this is a childhood cancer which initially develops in the kidneys. Patients typically present with a mass in the flank which is associated with haematuria.

4. **L. Renal calculus**

   The correct answer is renal calculus. Renal calculi are hard deposits that form within the kidney. Passage of stones can be quite painful; the pain is usually described as being in loin to groin distribution.

5. **F. Chronic prostatitis**

   The correct answer is chronic prostatitis. This is defined as prostatitis lasting more than three months. The pre-prostatic and post-prostatic massage test (PPMT), also known as the two-glass test, is diagnostic for chronic bacterial prostatitis if there are more than 20 leukocytes per high powered field on the post massage sample.

Musculoskeletal

7

ANKLE AND SHIN 1

A. Achilles tendinopathy
B. Achilles tendon rupture
C. Acute compartment syndrome
D. Anterior talo-fibular ligament injury
E. Charcot arthropathy
F. Chronic ankle instability
G. Deep vein thrombosis
H. Gastrocnemius tear
 I. Lateral process of the talus fracture
J. Navicular stress fracture
K. Osteoid osteoma
L. Post-Thrombotic syndrome
M. Shin splints
N. Sinus tarsi syndrome
O. Subtalar dislocation
P. Superficial thrombophlebitis
Q. Tibialis posterior rupture
R. Tibialis posterior tendinitis
S. Tibiofibular diastasis
T. Flexor hallucis longus tendonitis
U. Varicose veins

For each of the following, what is the MOST likely diagnosis?

1. A 35-year-old woman attends with left lower leg pain. The pain has been present for the past two days. She has no significant past medical history, is taking the oral contraceptive pill, is a non-smoker and has not recently travelled. On examination she has red swollen skin over the left calf and you palpate a tough cord-like vein under the surface of the affected skin. Pain is elicited by ankle flexion.

DOI: 10.1201/9781003459941-7

2. A 28-year-old hockey player complains of severe left shin pain. He was struck on the shin while playing an hour ago and has had progressively worsening pain and swelling. On examination the skin in the anterior shin appears stretched and shiny and is significantly tender to touch.

3. A 21-year-old man presents with acute pain in the back of his right leg and inability to ambulate on the affected side. He was out running and felt a sudden pop in the back of his leg followed by excruciating pain. On examination Thompson test is positive.

4. A 55-year-old diabetic presents with a three-month history of pain in his right lower limb. His leg feels heavy, the pain is worse with standing and better when resting or with elevation. He had a DVT two weeks ago and is compliant with all of his medications. On examination he has a temperature of 36.7°C, a heart rate of 76 beats per minute, the skin over his right lower limb appears a dark red color.

5. A 53-year-old type 2 diabetic presents with a 12-month history of progressively worsening right ankle pain. On examination the foot is swollen, there is collapse of the medial arch and rocker bottom deformity is present. He has reduced sensation across the entire ankle.

See page 178 for answers.

ANKLE AND SHIN 2

A. Achilles tendinopathy
B. Achilles tendon rupture
C. Acute compartment syndrome
D. Anterior talo-fibular ligament injury
E. Charcot arthropathy
F. Chronic ankle instability
G. Deep vein thrombosis
H. Gastrocnemius tear
 I. Lateral process of the talus fracture
 J. Navicular stress fracture
K. Osteoid osteoma
L. Post-Thrombotic syndrome
M. Shin splints
N. Sinus tarsi syndrome
O. Subtalar dislocation
 P. Superficial thrombophlebitis
Q. Tibialis posterior rupture

R. **Tibialis posterior tendinitis**
S. **Tibiofibular diastasis**
T. **Flexor hallucis longus tendonitis**
U. **Varicose veins**

For each of the following, what is the MOST likely diagnosis?

1. A 27-year-old woman attends with right foot pain. She is a hockey player and last night she was struck on the inner aspect of her foot by another player's stick, there was sudden pain and she felt a pop in her ankle. On examination there is swelling and bruising over the medial malleolus, there is a collapse of the arch of the foot, the heel is tilted outwards and on observation of the foot posteriorly the "too many toes" sign is obvious.

2. A 31-year-old cricket player attends with left calf pain. She explains that it started yesterday while training. She felt a sudden pain in the back of her leg "as though someone kicked me really hard", but when she turned around there was nothing behind her. Thompson test is negative and she has some swelling in the posteromedial aspect of her left calf.

3. A 27-year-old Olympian attends with a three-week history of bilateral dull pain over his shins. He has been struggling to take part in his regular training sessions as a result. On examination he has tenderness on palpation of the distal two-thirds of medial tibial border over the length of 7 cm.

4. An 8-year-old boy presents with his parents who are concerned about pain he has had in his left leg during the night for the past two weeks. His mother has been massaging his leg and giving him paracetamol but this has not helped much. The local pharmacist suggested the use of ibuprofen, this has been helpful.

5. A 41-year-old type 2 diabetic presents with left lower leg pain and he cannot ambulate due to the pain. He had surgery for a torn medial meniscus in his left leg two days ago. On examination the left calf is tender to palpation and swollen.

6. A 24-year-old presents with pain in her left ankle. She had an inversion injury while bushwalking five days ago. She is ambulating but finds it painful to do so. On examination there is bruising inferior to the lateral malleolus and associated tenderness to palpation. Anterior drawer test is positive.

See page 178 for answers.

BACK PAIN 1

A. **Ankylosing spondylitis**
B. **Brown–Sequard syndrome**
C. **Cauda equina syndrome**

D. Dissecting thoracic aneurysm

E. Episacral lipoma

F. Multiple myeloma

G. Musculoligamentous strain

H. Pancreatitis

I. Pyelonephritis

J. Renal calculus

K. Retroperitoneal hematoma

L. Rheumatoid arthritis

M. Sacroiliac joint dysfunction

N. Scheuermann's disease

O. Spina bifida occulta

P. Spinal abscess

Q. Spinal canal stenosis

R. Spinal compression fracture

For each of the following, what is the MOST likely diagnosis?

1. A 58-year-old man attends with central chest pain which started 20 minutes ago. The pain is "tearing" in nature and radiates through to his back. On examination he has a BP of 186/112 mmHg in his left arm and an absent right sided radial pulse.

2. A 55-year-old woman presents with a six-month history of sacroiliac joint pain. During this time, she has lost 5 kg. You arrange for pathology which reveals an ESR of 116 and significant urinary excretion of immunoglobulin light chains.

3. A 63-year-old woman attends with lower back pain. The pain is worse on walking and associated with numbness and heaviness in both lower limbs. Her symptoms are relieved when she sits down to rest or leans forward on her shopping cart.

4. A 41-year-old woman presents with a four-hour history of sudden onset of left sided back pain which radiates to her left groin. The pain is 10/10 and comes in waves. On examination she is writhing about in pain, has a temperature of 36.0°C, heart rate of 84 beats per minute and a BP of 122/90 mmHg. She is tender in the left flank. Urine dipstick reveals haematuria.

5. A 23-year-old male attends after he burnt his right leg on a hot water bottle which he left on his leg overnight. He recently attended the local A&E after a stab injury he received to the left side of his back one week ago and reports that he has "not been quite the same" since. He complains of weakness on the left side of his body which affect his lower limb and he has had a couple of episodes of urinary incontinence.

See page 179 for answers.

BACK PAIN 2

A. Ankylosing spondylitis
B. Brown–Sequard syndrome
C. Cauda equina syndrome
D. Dissecting thoracic aneurysm
E. Episacral lipoma
F. Multiple myeloma
G. Musculoligamentous strain
H. Pancreatitis
I. Pyelonephritis
J. Renal calculus
K. Retroperitoneal hematoma
L. Rheumatoid arthritis
M. Sacroiliac joint dysfunction
N. Scheuermann's disease
O. Spina bifida occulta
P. Spinal abscess
Q. Spinal canal stenosis
R. Spinal compression fracture

For each of the following, what is the MOST likely diagnosis?

1. A 29-year-old woman presents with a five-day history of worsening lower back pain. She has a history of anxiety and IV drug use. On examination she has a temperature of 38.3°C and is tender in her lumbar spine.
2. A 32-year-old man presents with a six-month history of lower back pain. His symptoms are worse when he wakes but improve throughout the day. He also has pain in his heels when he gets out of bed. On examination there is decreased forward flexion of the spine. You arrange an X-ray of his spine which reveals a bamboo spine appearance.
3. A 61-year-old woman presents with severe back pain after a gym session yesterday. During her session there was a new instructor who incorporated weight lifting into her routine, something she normally does not do. She is struggling to straighten her back and reports that she has a loss of sensation in her left big toe and pain at the back of her left thigh. She has a past history of depression, osteoporosis and familial hyperlipidaemia. On examination you confirm the sensory loss on her left great toe, she cannot fully extend her left toe and struggles with dorsiflexion of her left ankle.
4. A 14-year-old girl presents with back ache. She is concerned about her worsening posture. On examination she has marked thoracic kyphosis. An X-ray of the spine reveals anterior wedging of three thoracic vertebrae.
5. A 26-year-old woman presents with lower back pain and numbness in her lower limbs. Two days ago, she slipped down a flight of stairs, landed on her bottom

and felt a sudden shooting pain down her back. The pain has progressively worsened, she has had difficulty ambulating, has developed numbness in her legs today and had an episode of urinary incontinence this morning.

See page 179 for answers.

ELBOW AND FOREARM 1

A. **Cubital tunnel syndrome**
B. **De Quervain's tenosynovitis**
C. **Intersection syndrome**
D. **Lateral epicondylitis**
E. **Medial epicondylitis**
F. **Olecranon bursitis**
G. **Panner's disease**
H. **Posterior interosseus nerve syndrome**
 I. **Radial tunnel syndrome**
J. **Valgus extension overload syndrome**

For each of the following, what is the MOST likely diagnosis?

1. A 17-year-old baseball player attends with right elbow pain for the past week. The pain affects the posteromedial aspect of her elbow and maximal pain occurs just as she releases the ball while pitching. On examination she is tender over the posteromedial elbow on the right and her symptoms are reproduced by application of valgus stress on the elbow at 20 degrees of flexion while simultaneously forcing the elbow into extension. An X-ray reveals osteophyte formation in the posteromedial olecranon fossa.

2. A 32-year-old accountant presents with a three-month history of right forearm pain. Initially it only occurred while playing squash but it is now impacting her ability to work and perform household tasks. On examination there is swelling on the dorsum of the forearm 5 cm proximal to Lister's tubercle, there is also tenderness and crepitus over the site of irritation. She struggles to pronate her arm secondary to pain.

3. An 8-year-old boy presents with right lateral elbow pain for the past four weeks which has not improved. The pain is exacerbated by throwing balls when doing baseball training. On examination he has a full range of movement in the elbow and no obvious deformity. An X-ray reveals flattening of the capitellum.

4. A 29-year-old woman attends with a four-week history of left radial side wrist pain. She has a 6-month-old child and explains that the pain is worse when lifting her child. On examination there is swelling and tenderness over the first dorsal compartment of the left wrist. Finkelstein test is positive.

5. A 27-year-old athlete presents with pain on the medial aspect of his right elbow. The pain has been present for eight weeks and is associated with pins and needles on the medial side of his forearm and his 4th and 5th digits. On examination there is reduced sensation in the medial two fingers and Wartenberg's sign is positive.

See page 180 for answers.

ELBOW AND FOREARM 2

A. **Cubital tunnel syndrome**
B. **De Quervain's tenosynovitis**
C. **Intersection syndrome**
D. **Lateral epicondylitis**
E. **Medial epicondylitis**
F. **Olecranon bursitis**
G. **Panner's disease**
H. **Posterior interosseus nerve syndrome**
 I. **Radial tunnel syndrome**
J. **Valgus extension overload syndrome**

For each of the following, what is the MOST likely diagnosis?

1. A 22-year-old university student presents with weakness in his right hand and wrist. His symptoms have developed over recent months and he has found it difficult to write notes. You review his file and note that he has a two-year history of intermittent right elbow pain without a history of trauma. He has no other medical history. On examination he is unable to extend his fingers at the MCP joints and he has weak extension of his wrist, there is no loss of sensation.
2. A 32-year-old receptionist attends your clinic with left elbow pain. She knocked her elbow a few days ago after a fall and since then she has had worsening swelling over the elbow and associated pain. On examination you note swelling over the olecranon process which resembles a "goose egg" in appearance, there is tenderness on palpation over the site.
3. A 32-year-old man presents with pain in his right elbow for the past two weeks associated with a weak grip. He denies a history of trauma and has no significant past medical history other than anxiety. On examination there is swelling over the elbow and elbow pain is provoked by resisted extension of his wrist.
4. A 37-year-old carpenter presents with a six-month history of right lateral elbow pain. He reports that pain is worse when he is using a screwdriver or doing heavy lifting at work. On examination there is tenderness 5 cm distal to the lateral epicondyle, the pain is made worse with elbow extension, wrist flexion and forearm pronation. There is no sensory or motor deficit.

5. A 39-year-old woman presents with a three-month history of right elbow pain and swelling. She denies a history of trauma and has been well otherwise. On examination there is swelling in the elbow, there is also pain with resisted forearm pronation and wrist flexion.

See pages 180–181 for answers.

FOOT PAIN 1

A. Freiberg disease
B. Gout
C. Growing pain
D. Hallux valgus
E. Hammer toe
F. Heel fat pad syndrome
G. Kohler disease
H. Mallet toe
I. Morton's neuroma
J. Plantar fasciitis
K. Pseudogout
L. Sever's disease
M. Stress fracture
N. Talon noir
O. Tarsal tunnel syndrome

For each of the following, what is the MOST likely diagnosis?

1. A 37-year-old woman presents with a six-month history of pain in her left foot when she puts on her shoes. She denies any trauma and has no significant medical history. On examination she has hyperflexion of the distal interphalangeal joint of the third toe.
2. A 16-year-old girl presents with a ten-month history of left forefoot pain. On examination she has tenderness over the second metatarsophalangeal joint with associated swelling and restricted dorsiflexion. You arrange for an X-ray which reveals flattening of the second metatarsal head with subchondral sclerosis.
3. A 65-year-old man presents with a six-month history of right foot pain. The pain is mostly in the middle of his heel and feels deep and "bruise like". His pain is worse with walking and after prolonged periods of standing. On examination you are able to reproduce the pain with firm palpation over the heel. You arrange for an ultrasound which reveals a fat pad of 0.9 cm thickness (normal > 1.2 cm), but nil else.
4. A 43-year-old woman presents with a five-month history of right foot pain. The pain is in her heel and is worse first thing in the morning when she steps out of

bed but gradually improves with walking. She has a history of anxiety, ankylosing spondylitis and a bone spur at the base of her right foot. On examination she has point tenderness along the anteromedial calcaneum.

5. A 57-year-old man presents with a one-day history of right great toe pain and swelling. His pain is so severe that he is unable to walk using his right foot. He denies any trauma and has no significant medical history. He is a non-smoker and drinks eight standard drinks each weekend, he has done this for the past 15 years. On examination he has a temperature of 36.6°C, blood pressure of 126/84 mmHg, heart rate of 68 beats per minute, respiratory rate of 16 breaths per minute and a BMI of 34. You perform an aspiration of joint fluid from the toe, this reveals negatively birefringent needle like crystals.

See page 181 for answers.

FOOT PAIN 2

A. Freiberg disease
B. Gout
C. Growing pain
D. Hallux valgus
E. Hammer toe
F. Heel fat pad syndrome
G. Kohler disease
H. Mallet toe
I. Morton's neuroma
J. Plantar fasciitis
K. Pseudogout
L. Sever's disease
M. Stress fracture
N. Talon noir
O. Tarsal tunnel syndrome

For each of the following, what is the MOST likely diagnosis?

1. A 7-year-old boy attends your clinic with his parents who are very concerned. He woke up last night complaining of bilateral foot pain, his parents gave him paracetamol and massaged his feet which helped resolve his symptoms within 45 minutes. He has had similar episodes over the past two weeks. On examination you find no cause for his symptoms and he is walking about comfortably.

2. A 24-year-old woman presents with discoloration in her heel. She noticed black streaks in her left heel yesterday after basketball training. She denies any pain

or history of trauma. On examination there are two arrowhead shaped black macules measuring 7 mm and 9 mm respectively.

3. An 11-year-old boy presents with bilateral heel pain. He has been symptomatic for the past five months and it is worse after running. On examination there is swelling and significant tenderness at the back of both heels.

4. A 51-year-old man presents with discomfort and pain affecting his left foot. He has episodes of burning pain and numbness in the medial aspect of his foot extending into his great toe. He explains that his symptoms have been present for the past eight months. On examination Tinel's sign is positive.

5. A 64-year-old woman presents with a two-day history of left foot pain and swelling mostly affecting her great toe. She struggles to ambulate as a result of the pain. She denies trauma and has no significant medical history. She is a non-smoker and does not drink alcohol. On examination she has a temperature of 36.3°C, blood pressure of 136/90 mmHg, heart rate of 72 beats per minute, respiratory rate of 18 breaths per minute and a BMI of 30. You note significant swelling affecting her left great toe. You perform an aspiration of joint fluid from the toe, this reveals rod shaped crystals with blunt ends which are positively birefringent.

See pages 181–182 for answers.

FOOT PAIN 3

A. Freiberg disease
B. Gout
C. Growing pain
D. Hallux valgus
E. Hammer toe
F. Heel fat pad syndrome
G. Kohler disease
H. Mallet toe
 I. Morton's neuroma
J. Plantar fasciitis
K. Pseudogout
L. Sever's disease
M. Stress fracture
N. Talon noir
O. Tarsal tunnel syndrome

For each of the following, what is the MOST likely diagnosis?

1. A 28-year-old woman presents with pain in her right foot when she puts on her shoes. Her symptoms have been present for the past six months, she denies any trauma and has no significant medical history. On examination she has hyper-extension of her second metatarsophalangeal joint, flexion of the proximal interphalangeal joint and extension of the distal interphalangeal joint.

2. A 42-year-old woman presents with an eight-month history of right great toe pain. She explains that the pain has come about gradually and she has noticed that the skin on the medial aspect of her big toe has become thickened and red. On examination you note medial swelling over the great toe and lateral deviation of the toe.

3. A 28-year-old runner presents with pain in her right foot. She explains that the pain occurs between the third and fourth metatarsal space and is worse with running and walking. On examination Mulder's click test is positive.

4. A 7-year-old boy presents with his parents who explain that he has been complaining of arch pain affecting his left foot. The pain is worse after activity and at times causes him discomfort for several days after strenuous physical activity. On examination there is tenderness over the navicular bone. You organise an X-ray which reveals that the navicular bone has a wafer like appearance and fragmentation.

5. A 37-year-old woman presents with pain in the dorsum of her right foot for the past two days. She explains that she has recently started running and does so for most days of the week. She has no significant medical history. On examination she is tender over the shaft of the second metatarsal.

See page 182 for answers.

HAND AND WRIST 1

A. **Anterior interosseous syndrome**
B. **Carpal tunnel syndrome**
C. **Chilblains**
D. **Dupuytren's disease**
E. **Erythromelalgia**
F. **Guyon's canal syndrome**
G. **Hypothenar hammer syndrome**
H. **Haemochromatosis**
I. **Jaccoud arthropathy**
J. **Kienbock's disease**
K. **Median nerve palsy**
L. **Osteoarthritis**
M. **Psoriatic arthritis**
N. **Raynaud's disease**

O. **Rheumatoid arthritis**
P. **Scaphoid fracture**
Q. **Scapholunate ligament injury**
R. **Scleroderma**
S. **Systemic lupus erythematosus**
T. **Wartenberg's syndrome**

For each of the following, what is the MOST likely diagnosis?

1. A 29-year-old labourer has a painful nodule in his right palm which has been present for the past two months. The nodule has thickened with time and the ring finger is more flexed as a result. He is struggling with his work as a result of this condition. On examination there is a nodule in the medial aspect of the palm and Hueston's tabletop test is positive.

2. A 36-year-old woman presents with painful discoloration of her fingers. She first noticed her symptoms six months ago and reports that symptoms are made worse with cold weather. On questioning she also reports thickening of the skin around her hands and she has been suffering from dysphagia.

3. A 24-year-old figure skater presents with pain in her fingers. She reports that she has developed tender bumps in her fingers which are at times itchy. They appear mostly when she is outdoors on cold days or after ice skating sessions, lasting up to two days after onset. She has no significant medical history and is a smoker. On examination there are small blanching bumps across her fingers which are purple and red in color.

4. A 31-year-old chef attends with weakness in her hand for the past three weeks. She was at work and accidentally cut her wrist on a kitchen knife just prior to the onset of her symptoms. On examination you note that the thenar eminence appears flat, there is decreased ability to flex the lateral three digits and oppose the thumb.

5. A 39-year-old woman presents with a 3-month history of bilateral hand pain and wrist swelling. She explains that she has also had intermittent ankle and knee pain. She has no history of trauma. On examination you note swelling in the wrist and hands. You also note a butterfly rash across her face and nasal ulcers. You arrange for pathology which is negative for anti-CCP antibodies, negative for RF but positive for ANA and anti-dsDNA. She also has an eGFR of 49.

6. A 42-year-old woman presents with a 4-day history of pain in her left index and middle fingers. She has had no trauma and reports that her symptoms are affecting her daily activities. On examination her left index finger and middle finger are red and swollen with a sausage-like appearance.

See pages 182–183 for answers.

HAND AND WRIST 2

A. Anterior interosseous syndrome
B. Carpal tunnel syndrome
C. Chilblains
D. Dupuytren's disease
E. Erythromelalgia
F. Guyon's canal syndrome
G. Hypothenar hammer syndrome
H. Haemochromatosis
 I. Jaccoud arthropathy
 J. Kienbock's disease
K. Median nerve palsy
L. Osteoarthritis
M. Psoriatic arthritis
N. Raynaud's disease
O. Rheumatoid arthritis
P. Scaphoid fracture
Q. Scapholunate ligament injury
R. Scleroderma
S. Systemic lupus erythematosus
T. Wartenberg's syndrome

For each of the following, what is the MOST likely diagnosis?

1. A 16-year-old girl presents with worsening left wrist pain. She has had pain at the base of her thumb for the past two weeks after a fall on an outstretched hand while skateboarding She had an X-ray at the time of the fall and "the nurse told me that there weren't any broken bones so I left the emergency department because the doctor was taking so long to get to me". On examination there is wrist swelling laterally and there is tenderness on palpation of the anatomical snuff box.

2. A 56-year-old woman presents to your clinic complaining of bilateral hand pain and swelling. Her symptoms have been present for the past 12 months and are progressively worsening. She has no history of recent trauma and explains that the pain is worse at the end of the day. On examination there is swelling in the proximal interphalangeal (PIP) joints and distal interphalangeal (DIP) joints. You arrange an X-ray of her hands which reveals loss of joint spaces and osteophyte formation at the PIP and DIP joints.

3. A 19-year-old woman complains of painful color changes to her hands for the past two weeks. She reports that some of her fingers turn dark purple when exposed to the cold. She has no past medical history of note and does not use any regular medications. On examination you are able to reproduce the discoloration by giving her a cup of ice-cold water to hold. Furthermore, her skin is intact and she has no other physical findings.

4. A 52-year-old woman presents with a three-month history of wrist and ankle pain. She explains that her symptoms are worse in the morning and she has associated joint stiffness, which lasts for at least an hour, improving throughout the day. She has also been feeling fatigued. On examination she has no obvious deformity but has wrist and ankle tenderness on palpation.

5. A 37-year-old woman complains of a five-month history of progressively worsening bilateral hand pain with associated metacarpal-phalangeal joint swelling. She has no significant medical history and reports that her father passed away in his early 50s from heart failure. On examination there is tenderness over the joints of the hands bilaterally. You arrange an X-ray which demonstrates hook like osteophytes from the radial ends of the second and third metacarpals.

6. A 27-year-old woman presents to your clinic complaining of discomfort in her hands. She reports that she has been having episodes of numbness affecting the lateral three and a half fingers and decreased grip strength. Her symptoms are particularly worse at night and she feels relief when she hangs her hands over the edge of her bed. She has no significant past medical history and is currently 26 weeks gestation.

See pages 183–184 for answers.

HIP PAIN 1

A. Coxa saltans
B. Developmental dysplasia of hip
C. Ewing sarcoma
D. Femoroacetabular impingement
E. Inguinal hernia
F. Labral tear
G. Meralgia paraesthetica
H. Neck of femur fracture
I. Osteitis pubis
J. Perthes disease
K. Piriformis syndrome
L. Polymyalgia rheumatica
M. Slipped capital femoral epiphysis
N. Transient hip synovitis
O. Trochanteric bursitis

For each of the following, what is the MOST likely diagnosis?

1. A 56-year-old mechanic presents with a six-month history of pain in his right hip and groin. He explains that his symptoms are exacerbated by heavy lifting and as a result he has had to reduce his work hours. He has no significant medical history. On examination he has a positive cough impulse in the right groin.
2. A 53-year-old woman complains of right sided hip pain. She describes the pain as a deep ache which has been present for the past eight weeks and reports that direct contact over the outer surface of her hip is very painful. She explains that she is struggling to sleep at night as a result of her symptoms as she cannot lay on her right side. On examination her symptoms are reproduced by palpating the upper outer surface of her right thigh.
3. An 81-year-old woman presents with right hip pain. She was in her lounge room and tripped over her dog. On examination her right leg is shortened, abducted and externally rotated.
4. A 21-year-old athlete presents with a four-week history of deep pelvic pain. On examination the pain is reproduced by performing the pubic spring test. You arrange for an X-ray which reveals sclerosis and lysis around the pubic symphysis, you also note widening of the symphysis.
5. A 12-day-old is referred to your orthopedic outpatient clinic by her GP who is concerned about her left hip. Her mother explains that she is their first child and she had an uneventful vaginal delivery at term. On examination there are normal thigh folds, galeazzi sign is positive on the left side.

See page 184 for answers.

HIP PAIN 2

A. Coxa saltans
B. Developmental dysplasia of hip
C. Ewing sarcoma
D. Femoroacetabular impingement
E. Inguinal hernia
F. Labral tear
G. Meralgia paraesthetica
H. Neck of femur fracture
I. Osteitis pubis
J. Perthes disease
K. Piriformis syndrome
L. Polymyalgia rheumatica
M. Femoral neck fracture
N. Transient hip synovitis
O. Trochanteric bursitis

For each of the following, what is the MOST likely diagnosis?

1. A 5-year-old girl presents with her parents who are concerned about her refusal to bear weight on her right hip. Her parents have noticed her limping today and complaining of pain in the hip. She has not been unwell recently and has no history of trauma. On examination she is afebrile and she has her right leg held in flexion and external rotation. Her CRP and WCC were normal.

2. A 20-year-old cricket player presents with left groin discomfort. He explains that he has had pain, numbness and a burning sensation in the anterolateral thigh for the past 12 months which has gradually worsened over the past month. On examination he has a full range of movement in the hip, with reduced sensation over the anterolateral thigh.

3. An 11-year-old boy presents complaining of left hip pain for the past five weeks. Since last night his pain has been more severe and he has been unable to walk. On examination he has a reduced range of movement in the left hip and the patient is unable to stand on his left leg. You arrange for an X-ray and observe Trethowan's sign on the left hip.

4. A 77-year-old woman presents with worsening hip pain for the past three months. She reports that her hips are stiffening up and she struggles to ambulate as a result. During this time, she has also been suffering from bilateral shoulder pain and struggling to hang her clothes on the line. She has an ESR of 110 mm/h.

5. A 6-year-old boy presents with left hip pain. Through tears, he reports that the pain has been there for the past week but has been significantly bad today causing him much pain and difficulty walking. He has no history of trauma and is otherwise well. You arrange for an X-ray of the hips which reveals marked flattening of the left femoral head.

See pages 184–185 for answers.

KNEE PAIN 1

A. Anterior cruciate ligament tear
B. Fractured patella
C. Hoffa's fat pad impingement
D. Iliotibial band syndrome
E. Infrapatellar bursitis
F. Knee dislocation
G. Knee synovial plica syndrome
H. Medial collateral ligament injury
I. Meniscal tear
J. Osgood–Schlatter disease
K. Osteochondritis dissecans
L. Patellar tendinopathy

M. **Patellofemoral pain syndrome**
N. **Pes anserinus bursitis**
O. **Posterior cruciate ligament tear**
P. **Prepatellar bursitis**
Q. **Reiter's syndrome**
R. **Ruptured Baker's cyst**
S. **Semimembranosus tendinopathy**
T. **Septic arthritis**
U. **Sinding–Larsen–Johansson syndrome**

For each of the following, what is the MOST likely diagnosis?

1. A 16-year-old girl presents with acute pain in her right knee. She reports that while playing netball she twisted her knee while it was flexed and locked to the ground. She felt a crack in her knee and it immediately began to swell. On examination the anterior drawer test is positive.
2. A 21-year-old woman presents with severe pain affecting her right knee. She reports that she has had swelling and pain behind her right knee for the past two weeks but it has gradually worsened and today she felt a pop in the back of her knee with severe pain. On examination she has swelling in her right calf with associated warmth and tenderness to palpation. The right calf measures 1 cm greater than the left.
3. A 21-year-old long distance runner presents with lateral knee pain. Over the past four months he has been trying to increase his level of activity in preparation for an upcoming event. He explains that when he over-exerts himself, he feels pain on the lateral aspect of his right knee, which takes a few days to settle but keeps returning.
4. A 39-year-old carpenter complains of anterior knee pain. On examination there is swelling on the anterior of the knee the size of a grapefruit.
5. A 23-year-old basketball player attends your clinic with anterior knee pain. His pain limits his participation in his sporting activities. He reports that the pain is worse with jumping. On examination there is tenderness on palpation of the inferior pole of the patella.

See page 185 for answers.

KNEE PAIN 2

A. **Anterior cruciate ligament tear**
B. **Fractured patella**
C. **Hoffa's fat pad impingement**
D. **Iliotibial band syndrome**
E. **Infrapatellar bursitis**

F. **Knee dislocation**
G. **Knee synovial plica syndrome**
H. **Medial collateral ligament injury**
 I. **Meniscal tear**
 J. **Osgood –Schlatter disease**
K. **Osteochondritis dissecans**
 L. **Patellar tendinopathy**
M. **Patellofemoral pain syndrome**
N. **Pes anserinus bursitis**
O. **Posterior cruciate ligament tear**
 P. **Prepatellar bursitis**
Q. **Reiter's syndrome**
R. **Ruptured Baker's cyst**
 S. **Semimembranosus tendinopathy**
 T. **Septic arthritis**
U. **Sinding–Larsen–Johansson syndrome**

For each of the following, what is the MOST likely diagnosis?

1. A 28-year-old man presents with pain deep in his left knee. His symptoms started two weeks ago after he sustained a twisting injury to his knee while he was playing soccer. Since the injury he explains that sometimes his leg will not straighten and he has to move it about before he can use it properly.

2. A 21-year-old man presents with a swollen and painful right knee and ankle. His symptoms started three days ago and he reports that he has also been suffering from recurrent episodes of dysuria and conjunctivitis for the past four weeks. He reports that he has had multiple sexual partners in the past four weeks.

3. A 16-year-old girl presents with a six-week history of right knee pain. She is a long-distance runner. She explains that her pain is worse when going up and down stairs and when her knees are bent for a prolonged period. Last night she had significant discomfort when she was out with friends at the cinema.

4. A 13-year-old boy complains of a six-month history of right knee pain and tenderness over the tibial tuberosity. He explains that the pain is worse with running and improves with rest. On examination there is enlargement of the right tibial tubercle. An X-ray reveals fragmentation of the tibial tubercle.

5. A 23-year-old male is brought into your emergency department under police escort. He was involved in a high-speed motor vehicle accident after allegedly stealing a car. He now has pain and swelling in his left knee after striking it on the dashboard.

6. A 43-year-old man presents with acute left knee pain and swelling. He denies trauma and reports that he is otherwise well. He has a history of depression and IV drug use. On examination he has a temperature of 38.1°C, the left knee is swollen and red with pain on all movements.

See pages 185–186 for answers.

NECK AND SHOULDER PAIN 1

A. Acromioclavicular joint disruption
B. Acute myocardial infarction
C. Adhesive capsulitis
D. Anterior shoulder dislocation
E. Biceps tendinitis
F. Brachial plexus injury
G. Klippel–Feil syndrome
H. Long head of biceps rupture
 I. Long thoracic nerve palsy
 J. Polymyalgia rheumatica
K. Posterior shoulder dislocation
L. Supraspinatus tendon rupture
M. Shoulder impingement syndrome
N. SLAP tear
O. Sprengel deformity
P. Thoracic outlet syndrome
Q. Torticollis

For each of the following, what is the MOST likely diagnosis?

1. A 57-year-old man presents with left shoulder pain. The pain started two hours ago and radiates into his neck and jaw. He has no history of trauma and the pain is not exacerbated by palpation. He has a history of diabetes, hypertension and hyperlipidaemia. He drinks two standard drinks a day on weekends and has smoked 20 cigarettes a day for the past 40 years. On examination he appears pale and clammy.

2. A 26-year-old power-lifter presents with discomfort in his right shoulder. He was training yesterday and heard a pop in his arm followed by sharp anterior shoulder pain. On examination of his arm, you note a positive Popeye sign.

3. A 26-year-old boxer attends your clinic after a boxing match he had last night. He complains of shoulder and rib pain on the left side of his body. He reports that he has a reduced range of movement in the shoulder. On examination the serratus anterior strength test is positive.

4. A 55-year-old type 2 diabetic presents with left shoulder pain and stiffness. Her symptoms have been present for the past six months and are progressively worsening. On examination there is restriction in all ranges of movement.

5. A 36-year-old woman is brought into your A&E by ambulance with left shoulder pain. She was at home and sustained an electric shock from a faulty appliance, the force of the shock pushed her across the room and she has had difficulty moving her shoulder since. An X-ray of her shoulder demonstrates the light bulb sign.

See page 186 for answers.

NECK AND SHOULDER PAIN 2

A. Acromioclavicular joint disruption
B. Acute myocardial infarction
C. Adhesive capsulitis
D. Anterior shoulder dislocation
E. Biceps tendinitis
F. Brachial plexus injury
G. Klippel–Feil syndrome
H. Long head of biceps rupture
 I. Long thoracic nerve palsy
 J. Polymyalgia rheumatica
K. Posterior shoulder dislocation
L. Supraspinatus tendon rupture
M. Shoulder impingement syndrome
N. SLAP tear
O. Sprengel deformity
P. Thoracic outlet syndrome
Q. Torticollis

For each of the following, what is the MOST likely diagnosis?

1. A 56-year-old factory worker presents with acute shoulder pain. She was lifting some boxes and felt a sudden sharp pain in her right shoulder. On examination she is tender in the shoulder, she struggles with active abduction and requires assistance through the first 90° but has a full range of passive and active movements otherwise.

2. A 22-year-old baseball player presents with left anterior shoulder pain for the past two weeks. On examination Yergason's test is positive and there is pain on palpation over the bicipital groove.

3. A 72-year-old woman presents with bilateral shoulder pain. Her symptoms have been present for the past eight months and she struggles to change her clothes or brush her hair. She also reports chronic pelvic pain. You arrange for laboratory testing and note an ESR of 87.

4. A 10-year-old boy attends your surgery with his mother. He complains of neck pain which started earlier in the day when he woke up. The pain has become worse throughout the day. He denies any recent illness or trauma. On examination he struggles to turn his head to the left.

See page 186 for answers.

ANSWERS

Ankle and shin 1

1. P. Superficial thrombophlebitis
This is a swollen vein as a result of a blood clot, patients usually report erythema and pain over the affected vein which feels hardened on palpation.

2. C. Acute compartment syndrome
This is a condition in which there is acute increase in pressure within an osteofascial compartment. This is a medical emergency and requires urgent treatment to reduce the pressure within the swollen compartment.

3. B. Achilles tendon rupture
Thompson test involves squeezing the calf muscles while the patient is in a prone position, normally this causes plantar flexion. Absence of plantar flexion suggests rupture of the Achilles tendon.

4. L. Post-Thrombotic syndrome
This is a chronic condition which can develop in individuals who have had a deep vein thrombosis.

5. E. Charcot arthropathy
This is a condition which typically occurs in patients with uncontrolled diabetes and is a consequence of peripheral neuropathy.

Ankle and shin 2

1. Q. Tibialis posterior rupture
Most patients who present with this condition have a history of acute trauma; the mechanism of the trauma is usually forced eversion of the ankle. The too many toes sign is a common examination finding.

2. H. Gastrocnemius tear
Also known as a monkey muscle tear, patients typically describe a history of sudden intense calf pain. Treatment is usually conservative and non-surgical.

3. M. Shin splints
Also known as medial tibial stress syndrome, it is described as a recurrent dull ache along the lower two-thirds of the tibia. Patients typically report that symptoms are worse during exercise.

4. K. Osteoid osteoma
This condition is usually unilateral and severe, NSAIDs help to improve the pain but paracetamol offers little help.

5. G. Deep vein thrombosis
These result from the formation of a blood clot in the deep veins of the lower limb. Symptoms can include, pain, swelling and localised tenderness. This patient has recently had surgery to the affected limb which is a risk factor for DVT formation and this is the likely cause for their presentation.

6. D. Anterior talo-fibular ligament injury
This is the most commonly injured ligament in the ankle and results from an inversion injury to the ankle. The anterior drawer test is used to assess

the strength of the ATFL, it is best performed at days four to five after injury.

Back pain 1

1. D. Dissecting thoracic aortic aneurysm
Patients typically present with sudden onset chest pain with radiation to the back, classically described as "tearing" or "ripping". They may also present with shortness of breath, unilateral paralysis and unilateral diminished or absent pulses.

2. F. Multiple myeloma
This is a form of cancer which forms in plasma cells in the bone marrow.

3. Q. Spinal canal stenosis
In this condition the spinal canal narrows resulting in compression of the spinal cord and associated nerves. Patients can experience pain, loss of sensation and numbness.

4. J. Renal calculus
Renal calculi are hard deposits that form within the kidney. Passage of stones can be quite painful; the pain is usually described as being in loin to groin distribution.

5. B. Brown–Sequard syndrome
This is a neurological condition which results from injury to one side of the spinal cord. Patients typically have paralysis and weakness on the ipsilateral side of the body, they also have a loss of sensation for temperature and pain on the contralateral side of the body. Patients may also suffer from urinary and bowel incontinence.

Back pain 2

1. P. Spinal abscess
This is a rare presentation in which there is swelling in the spine as a result of a build-up of pus. Abuse of IV drugs is associated with a higher prevalence of spinal abscess formation.

2. A. Ankylosing spondylitis
This is an inflammatory condition which affects the spine and over time can cause the spine to fuse and appear bamboo like. Some patients may develop plantar fasciitis.

3. R. Spinal compression fracture
On examination this patient has evidence of compression at the L5 level. She is at particular risk given a history of osteoporosis.

4. N. Scheuermann's disease
This is a condition which affects the upper back, causing it to become more rounded and hunched in appearance.

5. C. Cauda equina syndrome
This a disorder of the spine which is considered a medical emergency, requiring urgent surgical intervention. It results from compression of the nerve roots in the lumbar spine which impairs sensation, movement and bladder control.

Elbow and forearm 1

1. **J. Valgus extension overload syndrome**
   Also known as javelin thrower's elbow or pitcher's elbow, this condition is commonly seen in overhead throwing athletes. This condition is characterised by pain in the posteromedial aspect of the elbow which is secondary to repetitive micro trauma. Plain radiograph typically reveals osteophyte formation in the posteromedial olecranon fossa.

2. **C. Intersection syndrome**
   Patients with this syndrome typically present with forearm pain and swelling 4–6 cm proximal to listers tubercle. Crepitus is a common finding; patients also find pronation of the forearm more difficult than supination.

3. **G. Panner's disease**
   This condition involves the flattening of the lateral part of the humeral condyle – known as the capitellum – and is secondary to avascular necrosis. This disease is commonly seen in children under the age of ten and particularly in individuals who throw balls, the dominant upper limb is usually affected. It must be distinguished from osteochondritis dissecans which occurs in children aged over ten years.

4. **B. De Quervain's tenosynovitis**
   This condition is most commonly caused by overuse of the wrist, lifting a child repetitively using thumbs as leverage is a common cause. Finkelstein test is a provocative test which is useful for the diagnosis of de Quervain's tenosynovitis.

5. **A. Cubital tunnel syndrome**
   This condition involves the entrapment of the ulnar nerve at the medial aspect of the elbow. Wartenberg's sign is not to be confused with Wartenberg's syndrome. The sign is a result of weakness of the palmar interosseus muscle, which is innervated by the ulnar nerve, and the unopposed actions of the digiti minimi and digitorum communis which are innervated by the radial nerve.

Elbow and forearm 2

1. **H. Posterior interosseus nerve syndrome**
   Unlike radial tunnel syndrome, this condition is always associated with motor dysfunction. Patients typically present with weakness of extensor muscles in the hand and forearm which is preceded by forearm pain.

2. **F. Olecranon bursitis**
   This is a common presentation affecting the elbow, it is most commonly caused by direct trauma (in this case a fall to the ground) or repeated small injuries.

3. **D. Lateral epicondylitis**
   Also known as "tennis elbow", this is a common overuse injury of the elbow. Patients commonly complain of pain over the lateral aspect of the elbow which is exacerbated by activities requiring resisted wrist extension.

4. I. Radial tunnel syndrome

This is a compressive neuropathy of the proximal interosseus nerve at the level of the radial tunnel. Unlike posterior interosseus nerve syndrome there is no motor deficit.

5. E. Medial epicondylitis

Also known as "golfer's elbow", this condition is an overuse injury of the elbow. The pain is localised on the medial aspect of the elbow and is exacerbated by resisted pronation of the forearm and flexion of the wrist.

Foot pain 1

1. H. Mallet toe

This patient has characteristic findings on examination. This condition affects the second, third and fourth toes.

2. A. Freiberg disease

This is a condition, most commonly seen in teenage girls, which presents with forefoot pain. It is as a result of osteochondrosis of metatarsal heads, the second metatarsal head is most commonly affected.

3. F. Heel fat pad syndrome

The symptoms are similar to plantar fasciitis but are usually unilateral. In this condition the pain is felt in the middle of the heel unlike plantar fasciitis in which the pain is located at the anterolateral aspect of the calcaneus. It is due to either acute or chronic damage to the heel and its fatty and fibrous tissues.

4. J. Plantar fasciitis

Patients with plantar fasciitis commonly complain of pain which is worse first thing in the morning, or after exercise. It is commonly associated with ankylosing spondylitis.

5. B. Gout

Examination of a fluid aspirate under polarised red light allows differentiation between gout and pseudogout. Urate crystals, seen in gout, are negatively birefringent and needle shaped. Whereas pseudogout has positively birefringent rhomboid shaped calcium phosphate crystals.

Foot pain 2

1. C. Growing pain

This type of pain typically occurs at night and is usually bilateral. It is usually benign and self-limiting, but pain can also typically resolve with paracetamol and massage.

2. N. Talon noir

Also known as calcaneal petechiae, this is a benign condition. The discoloration is a result of repetitive shearing forces and is commonly found in young athletes and basketball players in particular.

3. L. Sever's disease

Also known as calcaneal apophysitis, it results from recurrent microtrauma affecting the growth plates of the calcaneus. A combination of rest, simple analgesia, and strengthening exercises can resolve the majority of cases.

4. O. Tarsal tunnel syndrome

Tinel's sign at the tarsal tunnel is used to detect peripheral neuropathy involving the tibial nerve. Symptoms can be replicated by performing this test which includes lightly tapping at the tarsal tunnel.

5. K. Pseudogout

Examination of a fluid aspirate under polarised red light allows differentiation between gout and pseudogout. Calcium pyrophosphate crystals are positively birefringent and rhomboid shaped. Whereas gout has urate crystals which are needle shaped and negatively birefringent.

Foot pain 3

1. E. Hammer toe

This patient has characteristic findings on examination. This condition affects the second, third and fourth toes. The middle joint of the toe develops a deformity similar to that of a hammer.

2. D. Hallux valgus

This is a very common cause of foot pain. In this condition the affected great toe deviates laterally over a prolonged period. Patients may present with a bony prominence known as a bunion on the medial side of the toe.

3. I. Morton's neuroma

Mulder's click test is a clinical test which is used to assess for Morton's neuroma. Pain and an associated click can be produced by squeezing the metatarsal heads on either side of the neuroma together with one hand while putting pressure on the affected interdigital space with the other.

4. G. Kohler disease

This condition, also known as avascular necrosis of the navicular bone, results from damage to the navicular bone in young children. Patients typically present with foot pain and limping.

5. M. Stress fracture

The correct answer is stress fracture. These are small cracks or bruising within the affected bones and are usually caused by overuse. They commonly occur when individuals change their regular activities or increase the intensity of their physical activities.

Hand and Wrist 1

1. D. Dupuytren's disease

This is a disorder in which there is painful nodule formation and contracture of the digits which reduce hand function. A history of manual labour is associated with increased risk of Dupuytren's disease development.

2. R. Scleroderma

Scleroderma is an autoimmune condition which results in thickening of skin and connective tissue. Raynaud's phenomenon and dysphagia are common findings. Pneumonic to help remember CREST (calcinosis cutis, Raynaud phenomenon, esophageal dysmotility, sclerodactyly and telangiectasia).

3. C. Chilblains

Also known as perniosis, this condition results from inflammation of small blood vessels in the skin after exposure to cold environments. Patients typically report symptoms including discoloration, blistering, itch and pain.

4. K. Median nerve palsy

This patient has injured the median nerve, this can result in wasting of the thenar muscles and reduced function of the lateral three fingers, sensation can also be reduced laterally as a result.

5. S. Systemic lupus erythematosus

This patient meets the SLICC criteria for SLE; with synovitis of two or more joints, cutaneous manifestations, nasal ulceration, renal involvement as well as positive serology for ANA and anti-dsDNA. For diagnosis four criteria must be met with at least one clinical feature and one laboratory finding.

6. M. Psoriatic arthritis

This is an autoimmune condition which affects the joints. It typically affects those with psoriasis but in a small number of people the skin disease occurs after onset of arthritis. Dactylitis (sausage finger) is a common finding in patients with psoriatic arthritis.

Hand and Wrist 2

1. P. Scaphoid fracture

This type of fracture is most commonly caused by a fall on an outstretched hand. Avascular necrosis is a common complication of a scaphoid fracture, and repeat X-rays are essential seven to ten days after injury. Anatomical snuff box tenderness is a common exam finding.

2. L. Osteoarthritis

This patient has typical examination findings and radiological findings associated with osteoarthritis. Osteophytes at the PIP joints are known as Bouchard's nodes and those at the DIP joints are known as Heberden's nodes.

3. N. Raynaud's disease

Also known as primary Raynaud's phenomenon, this condition involves an exaggerated response to cold without a known underlying cause. Patients with this condition usually have no abnormal findings on serology or examination.

4. O. Rheumatoid arthritis

This is an autoimmune condition which mainly affects the joints. This is a symmetrical form of arthritis which usually presents with morning stiffness which lasts at least an hour and improves throughout the day.

5. H. Haemochromatosis

This is an inherited condition in which the body absorbs and stores more iron than required. Arthropathy affecting the hands is a common finding and this patient has classic radiological and physical examination findings. Her father also passed away from heart failure which is a cardiac complication of haemochromatosis.

6. B. Carpal tunnel syndrome

This is a common syndrome which involves compression of the median nerve as it travels through the wrist. Patients typically describe loss of sensation and function of the lateral fingers. Pregnancy is a common cause.

Hip pain 1

1. E. Inguinal hernia

This occurs due to a bulging of the intra-abdominal contents through an area of weakness in the lower abdominal wall. Activities which increase intra-abdominal pressure such as lifting, coughing and sneezing can exacerbate symptoms.

2. O. Trochanteric bursitis

This condition involves inflammation of the bursa over the greater trochanter. Patients typically describe pain in the outside of the hip and thigh which is usually worse when lying on the affected side.

3. H. Neck of femur fracture

This patient has had acute trauma and has typical physical exam features of a neck of femur fracture. The leg is shortened and externally rotates due to the pull of the short external rotators.

4. I. Osteitis pubis

This condition results from inflammation of the pubic symphysis and surrounding muscle insertions.

5. B. Developmental dysplasia of hip

The galeazzi test is used to assess for hip dislocation, a positive sign suggests congenital hip malformation. Other examinations for hip dysplasia include the Barlow and Ortolani maneuvers.

Hip pain 2

1. N. Transient hip synovitis

This is a common cause for limp in a child and is as a result of inflammation of the synovium of the hip joint. The differential of a septic arthritis would usually be associated with elevated inflammatory markers.

2. G. Meralgia paraesthetica

This condition results from compression of the lateral femoral cutaneous nerve (branch of the lumbar plexus providing sensation to the anterolateral aspect of the upper thigh) as it passes under (occasionally through) the inguinal ligament.

3. M. Slipped capital femoral epiphysis

Trethowan's sign is a radiological feature observed when Klein's line does not intersect the lateral part of the superior femoral epiphysis.

4. L. Polymyalgia rheumatica

This is an inflammatory condition which causes muscle pain and stiffness. This condition is more common in those over the age of 50 and women are more likely to develop it than men. The shoulders and the hips are common sites of discomfort and a raised ESR level may be present.

5. J. Perthes disease

This is a condition which affects the hips of children between the ages of four and ten. In this condition there is disruption in the blood flow to the head of the femur resulting in avascular necrosis of the affected area.

Knee pain 1

1. A. Anterior cruciate ligament tear

This patient has had a twisting injury to a flexed knee which is firmly grounded. A tear to the anterior cruciate ligament can cause a bleed in the knee (haemarthrosis) and immediate swelling in the affected knee.

2. R. Ruptured Baker's cyst

A Baker's cyst (popliteal synovial cyst) is an accumulation of fluid in the bursa of the knee joint. These can rupture causing fluid to leak down the lower limb into the calf. This can be very painful; examination usually reveals swelling and redness.

3. D. Iliotibial band syndrome

This is the most common cause of lateral knee pain in runners, it is caused by overuse.

4. P. Prepatellar bursitis

Also known as carpenter's knee, this condition involves inflammation of a fluid filled sac known as the prepatellar bursa which is located in the anterior knee between the patella and superficial skin.

5. L. Patellar tendinopathy

Also known as jumper's knee, this is a form of anterior knee pain. Clinical diagnosis relies on tenderness on palpation of the inferior pole of the patella.

Knee pain 2

1. I. Meniscal tear

This patient likely has a bucket handle tear of the meniscus. This is a full thickness tear that occurs in the medial meniscus causing it to displace centrally, resulting in the locking of the knee joint.

2. Q. Reiter's syndrome

Also known as reactive arthritis, this is the most common form of inflammatory polyarthralgia in young males. The condition is characterised by conjunctivitis, urethritis and joint inflammation. The mnemonic "can't see, can't pee, can't climb a tree" is helpful in remembering this condition. STIs such as chlamydia are common causes for this presentation.

3. M. Patellofemoral pain syndrome

Also known as runner's knee, this is a pain syndrome caused by overuse. This patient demonstrates the classic "movie sign". Treatment is usually conservative.

4. J. Osgood–Schlatter disease

This is a common cause for knee pain particularly in young males. It occurs as a result of inflammation at the site where the patellar tendon attaches to the tibia.

5. **O. Posterior cruciate ligament tear**
   Displacement of the tibia posteriorly on a fixed femur results in the rupture of the posterior cruciate ligament. This can occur when the knee strikes a dashboard in a motor vehicle accident. In sporting activities, the injury typically occurs when a hyper-flexed knee strikes the ground.

6. **T. Septic arthritis**
   This is an infection in the joint fluid and surrounding tissues.

Neck and Shoulder pain 1

1. **B. Acute myocardial infarction**
   This patient has many risk factors for cardiovascular disease and acute onset of symptoms.

2. **H. Long head of biceps rupture**
   Popeye sign results from the bulging of the biceps muscle belly when detached.

3. **I. Long thoracic nerve palsy**
   This is a condition which affects the shoulder and is characterised by reduced function and pain secondary to injury of the long thoracic nerve (such as from a blow to the ribs). The nerve supplies the serratus anterior muscle (also known as the boxer's muscle), loss of function in this muscle results in winging of the scapula.

4. **C. Adhesive capsulitis**
   Also known as frozen shoulder, in this condition there is a reduced ability to move the shoulder both actively and passively. Diabetes and thyroid disease are risk factors but most cases are idiopathic. The condition typically resolves on its own but may take months to years to do so.

5. **K. Posterior shoulder dislocation**
   In this injury the head of the humerus is forced posteriorly in internal rotation while the arm is abducted. Electrocution is a classic cause of this presentation.

Neck and Shoulder pain 2

1. **L. Supraspinatus tendon rupture**
   This patient has physical findings which are typical of this type of injury.

2. **E. Biceps tendinitis**
   This condition involves the inflammation of the tendinous part of the long head of the biceps as it travels within the bicipital groove.

3. **J. Polymyalgia rheumatica**
   This is an inflammatory condition which causes muscle pain and stiffness. This condition is more common in those over the age of 50 and women are more likely to develop it than men. The shoulders and the hips are common sites of discomfort and a raised ESR level may be present.

4. **Q. Torticollis**
   Also known as wry neck this occurs as a result of muscle spasms in the neck. It is a common cause of neck pain in young individuals.

Cardiology

8

CHEST PAIN 1

A. Angina pectoris
B. Da Costa's syndrome
C. Dissecting thoracic aortic aneurysm
D. Dressler's syndrome
E. Oesophageal rupture
F. Oesophageal spasm
G. Myocardial infarction
H. Pericarditis
 I. Pneumothorax
J. Pulmonary embolism
K. Slipping rib syndrome
L. Takotsubo cardiomyopathy
M. Tietze's syndrome

For each of the following, what is the MOST likely diagnosis?

1. A 27-year-old secretary presents with a one-day history of central chest pain. The pain does not radiate and came on suddenly, she also has mild shortness of breath. The pain is 7/10 at its worst. Her medical history is unremarkable and the only medication she takes is the oral contraceptive pill. On examination, she is comfortable, talking in full sentences, she has a blood pressure of 124/82 mmHg, heart rate of 112 beats per minute, oxygen saturation of 98% at room air and lungs are clear to auscultation. Calves are soft and non-tender.

2. A 68-year-old male presents complaining of episodes of central chest pain with radiation to his left arm. He explains that the symptoms started a week ago, last about two to three minutes and are relieved by rest. He has a history of ischemic heart disease, hyperlipidaemia and hypertension. He is currently using aspirin, atorvastatin and perindopril. He has had no recent medication changes and reports that he is otherwise well.

3. You are a medical doctor supervising a local basketball competition, you are called urgently to the courtside just before halftime. A 21-year-old player

complains of sudden onset right sided chest pain associated with shortness of breath; he tells you that the pain is worse with inspiration. He denies trauma.

4. A 39-year-old woman presents with a six-month history of sudden, sharp, non-exertional central chest pain, associated with dysphagia of solids and fluids. The episodes last for about one to two minutes and then spontaneously resolve. You arrange for a barium swallow which reveals a corkscrew appearance.

See page 203 for answers.

CHEST PAIN 2

A. Angina pectoris
B. Da Costa's syndrome
C. Dissecting thoracic aortic aneurysm
D. Dressler's syndrome
E. Oesophageal rupture
F. Oesophageal spasm
G. Myocardial infarction
H. Pericarditis
 I. Pneumothorax
 J. Pulmonary embolism
K. Slipping rib syndrome
L. Takotsubo cardiomyopathy
M. Tietze's syndrome

For each of the following, what is the MOST likely diagnosis?

1. A 47-year-old man presents complaining of central chest pain. He explains that it started earlier in the day. The pain is described as sharp in nature and worse when lying down or taking a big breath in, he finds relief when sitting forward and also while exhaling. He had an upper respiratory tract infection five days ago but has been otherwise well.

2. A 61-year-old woman attends ED complaining of central chest pain which started 20 minutes ago, her daughter who attends with her explains that she described the pain initially as a tearing type pain which was radiating into her back. On examination she has a blood pressure of 202/116 in her left arm and an absent right sided radial pulse.

3. A 48-year-old electrician presents with left sided chest pain for the past three days. He has had no recent illness and no history of trauma. The pain is sharp and intermittent initially then becomes constant and can last for several hours at a time. The pain is in the lower ribs on the left side and there is a significant tenderness on palpation of a spot over the costal margin.

4. A 71-year-old male presents to your emergency department complaining of central chest pain radiating to his left arm. He describes the pain as severe and constant and it started 30 minutes ago. He tried sublingual GTN at home and after the third dose he contacted the ambulance service. On examination he is diaphoretic, has a regular pulse of 114, blood pressure of 162/96, temperature of 36.1°C, respiratory rate of 20 and saturations of 96% at room air. He has a history of IHD, angina, hyperlipidaemia and hypertension. You perform an ECG which reveals ST elevation in leads II, III and AVF.

See page 203 for answers.

CARDIAC VESSELS

A. **Coronary sinus**
B. **Great cardiac vein**
C. **Left anterior descending artery**
D. **Left circumflex artery**
E. **Left marginal vein**
F. **Left posterior ventricular vein**
G. **Middle cardiac vein**
H. **Right coronary artery**
I. **Superior vena cava**
J. **Small cardiac vein**

For each of the following, what is the MOST likely vessel affected?

1. A 53-year-old truck driver presents with left jaw pain and shoulder pain, this started 45 minutes ago. He has associated shortness of breath and is diaphoretic. You perform and ECG which reveals ST elevation in leads I, aVL, V5 and V6.
2. A 73-year-old type 2 diabetic presents with worsening shortness of breath and epigastric discomfort, she reports that it started one hour ago and is worsening, she has no associated chest pain. You perform an ECG which reveals ST elevation in leads V1, V2, V3 and aVR.
3. A 46-year-old presents to your emergency department complaining of sudden onset central chest pain which started 30 minutes ago, he reports that it radiates to his left jaw and arm. He has a history of hyperlipidaemia and hypertension. You perform an ECG which reveal ST elevation in leads II, III and aVF.

See page 203 for answers.

COLLAPSE 1

A. Addisonian crisis
B. Cardiac tamponade
C. Diabetic neuropathy
D. Epileptic seizure
E. Hypertrophic cardiomyopathy
F. Hypoglycaemia
G. Panic attack
H. Pulmonary embolism
 I. Stokes–Adams attack
J. Subclavian steal syndrome
K. Vasovagal syncope

For each of the following, what is the MOST likely diagnosis?

1. A 49-year-old type 2 diabetic woman presents complaining that she is feeling dizzy and has been collapsing at home. She has a history of hypertension and hyperlipidaemia. She is currently taking amlodipine, rosuvastatin, metformin and glimepiride. On examination she has a seated blood pressure of 148/96 mmHg and a standing blood presssure of 102/74 mmHg, you examine her feet and note sensory loss throughout. You review her most recent bloods and note that her HbA1c was 10.6 when measured last month and 10.2 three months earlier.

2. A 38-year-old flight attendant presents with shortness of breath and chest pain in your waiting room and then collapses and goes into cardiac arrest. She has no significant medical history and is currently using the oral contraceptive pill. Her partner explains that she returned home on a long-haul flight yesterday.

3. A 47-year-old woman is brought into your emergency department after fainting at the local pharmacy. She appears confused on arrival with slurred speech. Her husband is with her and explains that she has a history of type 2 diabetes and anxiety. She is using metformin, gliclazide, insulin and citalopram. Her GP added insulin to her management two days ago as her HbA1c readings were high. She took her diabetes medications this morning but had run out of her citalopram and left home before breakfast to run a few errands and collect her script from the pharmacy.

4. A 38-year-old man presents with a ten-day history of repeated episodes of syncope and associated fatigue. He explains that he has struggled to get out of his bed during this time. On examination you note that he has palmar hyperpigmentation, a blood pressure of 88/68 mmHg and he has a heart rate of 118 beats per minute. He has a finger prick BSL of 3.6. You arrange for laboratory investigations which reveal hyponatraemia and hyperkalaemia.

See page 204 for answers.

COLLAPSE 2

A. Addisonian crisis
B. Cardiac tamponade
C. Diabetic neuropathy
D. Epileptic seizure
E. Hypertrophic cardiomyopathy
F. Hypoglycaemia
G. Panic attack
H. Pulmonary embolism
 I. Stokes–Adams attack
J. Subclavian steal syndrome
K. Vasovagal syncope

For each of the following, what is the MOST likely diagnosis?

1. A 35-year-old woman presents with central chest pain and shortness of breath. She has a history of stage 4 breast cancer, hypothyroidism and Gilbert's syndrome. While you are talking to her she collapses and becomes unresponsive. On examination she has a blood pressure of 68/50 mmHg, muffled heart sounds and her JVP rises on inspiration.

2. A 36-year-old woman just returned from a short distance interstate flight and while at the luggage collection area she felt dizzy and collapsed to the floor. She explains that she suddenly noticed her heart begin to race, she felt tightness in her chest and reports that she felt short of breath. She remained conscious throughout and her symptoms have now resolved. She has no significant medical history. On examination you find no cause for her symptoms and her laboratory investigations are normal.

3. You are in the middle of a consult when your practice nurse enters your room in a hurry explaining that a 56-year-old man collapsed to the ground. You enter the waiting room where you find the man unresponsive and shaking uncontrollably. He recovers after three minutes and reports that he is very disorientated. During the episode he lost control of his bladder.

4. A 21-year-old male athlete presents to your emergency department after a collapse while he was running at a training session. There were no preceding symptoms and he has no significant medical history. He reports that his father passed away suddenly when he was aged 41. On examination there is a high pitched, mid-systolic, crescendo-decrescendo murmur over the left sternal border. The murmur does not radiate to the carotids.

5. A 32-year-old male attends your clinic for his pertussis vaccination. His wife is pregnant and their child is due shortly. You administer the vaccination, a few minutes later he appears pale and sweaty and explains that he feels dizzy. Before you can get him onto a chair he collapses to the ground. He is breathing and you palpate his pulse which is 42 beats per minute.

See page 204 for answers.

ARRHYTHMIAS 1

A. Acute pericarditis
B. Atrial fibrillation
C. Atrial flutter
D. Cardiac tamponade
E. First-Degree heart block
F. Hyperkalaemia
G. Hypertrophic cardiomyopathy
H. Pulmonary embolism
 I. Right bundle branch block
 J. Second-Degree heart block – Mobitz type 1
K. Second-Degree heart block – Mobitz type 2
L. Supraventricular tachycardia
M. Third-Degree heart block
N. Ventricular ectopic
O. Ventricular fibrillation
P. Ventricular tachycardia
Q. Wolff–Parkinson–White syndrome

For each of the following, what is the MOST likely diagnosis?

1. A 31-year-old woman presents after a road accident, complaining of central chest pain and shortness of breath. She has no significant medical history and is a non-smoker. On examination she has a blood pressure of 92/58 mmHg, muffled heart sounds and her JVP rises on inspiration. You attach an ECG which reveals sinus tachycardia and electrical alternans.

2. A 32-year-old woman presents with palpitations. She has no significant past medical history. You review her ECG which reveals shortened PR intervals and wide QRS complexes which are associated with slurred upstroke in lead II.

3. A 24-year-old presents for a pre-employment medical. He has no significant medical history and takes no regular medications. He examines well and is asymptomatic, on review of his ECG you note a prolonged PR interval.

4. A 71-year-old woman attends with intermittent palpitations for the past three days. On examination she has a blood pressure of 132/88 mmHg and a heart rate of 132 beats per minute. You arrange an ECG which reveals absent P waves and irregular QRS complexes.

5. A 34-year-old woman presents to your clinic with a three-week history of intermittent chest pain. You perform an ECG which reveals an RSR pattern in leads V1–V3 and a widened, slurred S wave in lead V6.

6. A 34-year-old man attends your clinic for a yearly work medical. He is asymptomatic today and denies any recent illness. He has no significant medical

history and takes no regular medication. You perform an ECG which reveals intermittent non conducted P waves without PR interval prolongation.

See pages 204–205 for answers.

ARRHYTHMIAS 2

A. **Acute pericarditis**
B. **Atrial fibrillation**
C. **Atrial flutter**
D. **Cardiac tamponade**
E. **First-Degree heart block**
F. **Hyperkalaemia**
G. **Hypertrophic cardiomyopathy**
H. **Pulmonary embolism**
I. **Right bundle branch block**
J. **Second-Degree heart block – Mobitz type 1**
K. **Second-Degree heart block – Mobitz type 2**
L. **Supraventricular tachycardia**
M. **Third-Degree heart block**
N. **Ventricular ectopic**
O. **Ventricular fibrillation**
P. **Ventricular tachycardia**
Q. **Wolff–Parkinson–White syndrome**

For each of the following, what is the MOST likely diagnosis?

1. A 29-year-old presents with a six-hour history of central chest pain. He reports that his pain is continuous, does not radiate and improves with expiration. He has no past medical history other than the common cold he recently had, which resolved two days ago. On examination he has a temperature of 36.9°C, heart rate of 102 beats per minute and a blood pressure of 128/78 mmHg. You arrange an ECG which reveals widespread concave ST elevation and PR depression in leads I, II, III, aVL, aVF and V2–V6. There is also ST depression and PR elevation in lead aVR and V1.

2. A 22-year-old university student presents to your clinic for review. She had a collapse yesterday while she was on her treadmill at home, she is unsure how long she was passed out for but did not feel the need to go to the local emergency department. There were no preceding symptoms and she has no significant medical history. She reports that her father passed away suddenly when he was aged 36. You perform an ECG which reveals large dagger like septal Q waves in the lateral and inferior leads.

3. A 56-year-old male presents with sudden onset central chest pain associated with lightheadedness and overwhelming fatigue. On physical examination at the time, he appeared comfortable, his blood pressure was 134/92 mmHg, oxygen saturation 98% room air, respiratory rate 20, heart rate 36 beats per minute and he had a temperature of 36.8°C. You perform an ECG and find that he has AV dissociation, he has an atrial rate of 100 and a ventricular rate of 36.

4. A 32-year-old woman presents with intermittent episodes of palpitations over the past week. She has a past medical history significant for anxiety and asthma. She uses salbutamol PRN and has no allergies. She reports that she is currently having an episode which started while in the wait room, you perform an ECG which reveals a regular narrow complex tachycardia at 190 beats per minute.

5. A 26-year-old librarian presents with central chest pain and shortness of breath. Her symptoms started earlier this morning and have been worsening. She has a history of polycystic ovarian syndrome and is on the combined oral contraceptive. On examination she has a heart rate of 112 beats per minute and a blood pressure of 132/84 mmHg. You perform an ECG which reveals sinus tachycardia, narrow QRS complexes and retrograde P waves.

See page 205 for answers.

HYPERTENSION 1

A. **Acromegaly**
B. **Aortic coarctation**
C. **Cushing syndrome**
D. **Hypothyroidism**
E. **Obstructive sleep apnoea**
F. **Phaeochromocytoma**
G. **Polycystic kidney disease**
H. **Primary hyperaldosteronism**
I. **Renal artery stenosis**
J. **Scleroderma renal crisis**

For each of the following, what is the MOST likely diagnosis?

1. A 43-year-old baggage handler reports that he has been feeling very fatigued for the past four months. He reports that he sleeps for ten hours but does not wake up feeling refreshed and often takes naps during the day. He explains that his wife complains that he snores loudly. On examination he has a weight of 122 kg, height of 171 cm, blood pressure 158/98 mmHg and a neck circumference of 42 cm.

2. A 36-year-old man attends for review of persistent hypertension. You notice on his file that he has been managed for hypertension for the past three years with multiple agents and limited success. His blood pressure today is 168/95 mmHg. He has no other significant medical history and is currently using an ACE inhibitor, a calcium channel blocker and a thiazide diuretic. You review his most recent bloods taken last week and note that he has a potassium of 3.0, he had been commenced on potassium supplements by his regular GP to treat this.

3. A 68-year-old woman presents for a general checkup. She has a history of hypertension, peripheral vascular disease, recurrent episodes of flash pulmonary edema and hyperlipidemia. She is currently taking atorvastatin, perindopril, amlodipine and hydrochlorothiazide. On examination she has a standing blood pressure of 158/86 mmHg and a seated blood pressure of 160/88 mmHg, she has a bruit on auscultation over the abdominal aorta.

4. A 48-year-old woman presents with fatigue, weight gain and weakness. On examination she has a heart rate of 86 beats per minute, a blood pressure of 158/98 mmHg, you note muscle wasting in her arms and legs, abdominal obesity, she has a rounded face and abdominal striae. You arrange for a dexamethasone suppression test which fails to reduce plasma cortisol following low dose dexamethasone administration.

See page 206 for answers.

See page 206 for answers.

HYPERTENSION 2

A. Acromegaly
B. Aortic coarctation
C. Cushing syndrome
D. Hypothyroidism
E. Obstructive sleep apnoea
F. Phaeochromocytoma
G. Polycystic kidney disease
H. Primary hyperaldosteronism
 I. Renal artery stenosis
J. Scleroderma renal crisis

For each of the following, what is the MOST likely diagnosis?

1. A 36-year-old male presents with a complaint of a severe headache associated with epistaxis. He has had intermittent headaches similar to this for the past three months. He has no significant medical history, takes no regular medications and smokes ten cigarettes a day which he has done since the age of 18. On examination he has a blood pressure of 206/108 and decreased femoral pulses.

2. A 41-year-old woman presents for a general check-up. She has no significant medical history and does not smoke or drink. On examination she has a blood pressure of 168/91 mmHg, there are palpable masses in bilateral flanks and mild hepatomegaly. Urine dipstick reveals hematuria.

3. A 37-year-old male attends with chronic headaches and worsening weakness in his hands. He tells you that he has been suffering from an early morning headache for the past two months. On examination he has a blood pressure of 156/94 mmHg, you note an enlarged head with frontal bossing and deep facial folds, he has enlarged hands and atrophy over bilateral thenar eminences.

4. A 46-year-old truck driver presents complaining of fatigue. He reports that he has gained 4 kg in weight over the past three months and has been suffering from constipation. On examination he has dry skin, a blood pressure of 154/102 mmHg, a heart rate of 56 beats per minute and has a BMI of 38. He has an elevated TSH and a reduced T4.

See page 206 for answers.

MURMURS 1

A. Aortic regurgitation
B. Aortic stenosis
C. Atrial myxoma
D. Coarctation of the aorta
E. Mitral regurgitation
F. Mitral stenosis
G. Patent ductus arteriosus
H. Pericarditis
 I. Pulmonary regurgitation
 J. Tricuspid regurgitation
K. Tricuspid stenosis

For each of the following, what is the MOST likely diagnosis?

1. A 43-year-old man presents for pre-operative assessment prior to an inguinal hernia repair next week. On examination de Musset's sign is positive and on auscultation of the praecordium you note a soft, high pitched, early diastolic decrescendo murmur which is loudest at the left sternal border at the level of the 3rd intercostal space. The sound is increased in intensity when he is sitting upright, leaning forward and asked to hold his breath in full expiration. Corrigan's pulse is visible at the carotids.

2. A 27-year-old woman presents with worsening shortness of breath associated with palpitations. On examination you hear a "tumor plop" during diastole on auscultation.

3. A 47-year-old woman complains of worsening shortness of breath and exercise dyspnoea. Her symptoms have been present for the past four months and are not improving. On examination her lungs are clear, on auscultation of the praecordium you note a high-pitched blowing holosystolic murmur, which is heard best at the apex and when the patient is in left lateral decubitus position. The murmur radiates through to the axilla and into the back. Carvallo's sign is absent and the sound of the murmur is decreased by Valsalva.

4. A 58-year-old woman attends for a pre-work medical assessment. She has been well and has a medical history significant for rheumatic heart disease. On auscultation of the praecordium you note a low-pitched diastolic rumble preceded by an opening snap, it is heard best at the 5th intercostal space on the midclavicular line. She examines well otherwise.

See page 207 for answers.

MURMURS 2

A. **Aortic regurgitation**
B. **Aortic stenosis**
C. **Atrial myxoma**
D. **Coarctation of the aorta**
E. **Mitral regurgitation**
F. **Mitral stenosis**
G. **Patent ductus arteriosus**
H. **Pericarditis**
I. **Pulmonary regurgitation**
J. **Tricuspid regurgitation**
K. **Tricuspid stenosis**

For each of the following, what is the MOST likely diagnosis?

1. A 58-year-old male presents to your clinic complaining of a pulsing sensation in his neck and abdominal swelling which have been present for the past few weeks. On examination of the neck, you note giant jugular "CV" waves. On auscultation of the praecordium you hear a high pitched, holosystolic, blowing murmur which is louder with deep inspiration. The murmur is heard best at the left lower sternal border. Abdominal examination reveals a pulsatile liver.

2. A 56-year-old woman presents with worsening fatigue and palpitations for the past six months. She has a history of pulmonary hypertension. On examination she has normal radial and carotid pulses. On auscultation of the praecordium you hear a decrescendo diastolic murmur with a blowing character, which is best heard on the upper left sternal border at the level of the second intercostal space.

3. A 6-year-old boy presents with a three-day history of chest pain. The pain is worse with inspiration and improves with leaning forward. On examination he

has a temperature of 38.5°C, a heart rate of 142 beats per minute, on auscultation of his chest there is a friction rub over Erb's point.

4. A 42-year-old woman presents with a three-week history of fatigue and fluttering discomfort in her neck. She reports that she has had abdominal swelling. On examination of her jugular veins, you note a giant flickering A wave with associated gradual y descent. On auscultation of the praecordium you hear a soft opening snap and mid diastolic rumble with presystolic accentuation.

See pages 207–208 for answers.

CHA$_2$DS$_2$-VASC SCORING

A. CHA$_2$DS$_2$-VASc score 0
B. CHA$_2$DS$_2$-VASc score 1
C. CHA$_2$DS$_2$-VASc score 2
D. CHA$_2$DS$_2$-VASc score 3
E. CHA$_2$DS$_2$-VASc score 4
F. CHA$_2$DS$_2$-VASc score 5
G. CHA$_2$DS$_2$-VASc score 6
H. CHA$_2$DS$_2$-VASc score 7

For the following patients with Atrial fibrillation please select the correct CHA$_2$DS$_2$-VASc score.

1. An 82-year-old man with a history significant for hypertension, congestive cardiac failure, hyperlipidaemia, GORD and benign prostate hypertrophy. His current medications include perindopril, atorvastatin, frusemide and prazosin. He is a non-smoker.
2. A 74-year-old woman with a history of hypertension and depression. Her only medication is captopril. She is a lifelong smoker.
3. A 35-year-old male with a history significant for diet-controlled type 2 diabetes mellitus and moderate mitral stenosis, he takes no regular medications.
4. A 58-year-old woman with a history of peripheral artery disease and hyperlipidaemia. She is currently taking atorvastatin and aspirin. She is a lifelong smoker and continues to smoke 20 cigarettes a day.
5. A 76-year-old diabetic trans male with a history of hypertension and previously had a provoked DVT after a long-haul flight. He is a non-smoker.

See page 208 for answers.

HYPERTENSION GRADING

A. **Optimal**
B. **Normal**
C. **High-Normal**
D. **Grade 1 (mild) hypertension**
E. **Grade 2 (moderate) hypertension**
F. **Grade 3 (severe) hypertension**
G. **Isolated systolic hypertension**

For each of the following select what best describes the blood pressure measurement.

1. A 22-year-old athlete is due to compete in a track event in a week and has attended for a medical assessment. She is asymptomatic on review. You perform a blood pressure measurement which reads 157/82 mmHg.
2. A 54-year-old man attends your clinic for a routine checkup. On examination he has a blood pressure which reads 118/72 mmHg.
3. A 67-year-old woman has been suffering from headaches which have been bothering her for the past three months. As part of your assessment, you perform a blood pressure measurement which reads 168/112 mmHg.
4. A 56-year-old diesel mechanic attends for repeat scripts for his asthma medication. He has been using Ventolin PRN and an inhaled corticosteroid to good effect and has had no adverse side effects. While in your consulting room you measure his blood pressure which reads 143/86 mmHg.
5. A 31-year-old fitness instructor attends your clinic for a workplace medical. As part of the examination, you take her blood pressure which measures 127/83 mmHg.

See page 208 for answers.

HEART FAILURE GRADING

A. **NYHA Class I**
B. **NYHA Class II**
C. **NYHA Class III**
D. **NYHA Class IV**
E. **NYHA Class V**

For each of the following select what best describes the patients' symptoms.

1. A 57-year-old male attends your clinic for a repeat script, he has a known history of congestive cardiac failure. He complains of a long history of shortness

of breath, this occurs at rest and gets worse with physical exertion. He reports that his symptoms have not acutely changed in the past few months.

2. A 68-year-old lady with a known history of congestive cardiac failure reports that she is comfortable at rest. She has been finding that she is slightly short of breath on exertion over the past few months but the symptoms resolve a few minutes after she rests. She is still very active and able to continue on with most of her activities of daily living.

3. A 74-year-old lady with a known history of congestive cardiac failure reports that she is comfortable at rest. She has been finding that she is increasingly short of breath on exertion over the past few months. Her symptoms have had a significant impact on her daily activities and she finds that she is struggling to walk more than a few meters before she is out of breath and has to stop.

See page 209 for answers.

CARDIAC STRUCTURE 1

A. **Atrial septal defect**
B. **Coarctation of the aorta**
C. **Dilated cardiomyopathy**
D. **Ebstein's anomaly**
E. **Hypertrophic cardiomyopathy**
F. **Hypoplastic left heart syndrome**
G. **Mitral valve prolapse**
H. **Patent ductus arteriosus**
I. **Peripartum cardiomyopathy**
J. **Restrictive cardiomyopathy**
K. **Tetralogy of Fallot**
L. **Transposition of the great arteries**
M. **Ventricular septal defect**

For each of the following, what is the MOST likely diagnosis?

1. A 34-year-old male attends for a railroad medical. He has no significant past medical history and takes no regular medication. On auscultation of the praecordium you note a widely split and fixed second heart sound. There is also a systolic murmur heard best at the upper left sternal border.

2. A newborn with Down syndrome attends your clinic with her mother for her six-week check, she was born via vaginal delivery and her mother has had an uneventful pregnancy. She is feeding well and her mother has no significant concerns. On auscultation of the praecordium there is a harsh pansystolic murmur at the left lower sternal edge, there is also a left parasternal heave.

3. A 36-year-old G5P4 woman presents at 32 weeks' gestation complaining of shortness of breath. She has a past history of bipolar disorder and has not been on any regular medications. On examination you auscultate crackles at bilateral bases of her lungs and she has pitting edema to the level of her knees bilaterally. You treat her for her symptoms and arrange for an echocardiogram which reveals an ejection fraction of 28%.

4. A 54-year-old woman presents with worsening shortness of breath. Her symptoms are exacerbated by exertion and she has also noticed swelling in her feet. She has a history of asthma and uses Ventolin regularly. She is a non-smoker; she drinks a bottle of wine a night and has done so for the past five years since her divorce. On examination she has pitting edema in bilateral lower limbs to the level of her ankles, on auscultation of the praecordium you note a third heart sound.

5. A 2-day-old child has been admitted to the paediatric ward with cyanosis since birth. On examination of the praecordium you hear a single loud second heart sound and a systolic ejection murmur. A chest X-ray reveals cardiomegaly with cardiac contours appearing like an egg on string.

See page 209 for answers.

CARDIAC STRUCTURE 2

A. Atrial septal defect
B. Coarctation of the aorta
C. Dilated cardiomyopathy
D. Ebstein's anomaly
E. Hypertrophic cardiomyopathy
F. Hypoplastic left heart syndrome
G. Mitral valve prolapse
H. Patent ductus arteriosus
 I. Peripartum cardiomyopathy
 J. Restrictive cardiomyopathy
K. Tetralogy of Fallot
L. Transposition of the great arteries
M. Ventricular septal defect

For each of the following, what is the MOST likely diagnosis?

1. A 24-year-old woman presents for a pre-work assessment. She is asymptomatic and reports that she has no significant medical history. On auscultation of the praecordium you hear a mid-systolic click which is best heard at the apex in left lateral decubitus position.

2. A 25-year-old woman presents for antenatal care. She is currently at 18 weeks' gestation and this is her first appointment with a doctor. She has a history of bipolar disorder and is currently being treated with lithium. You arrange for a fetal ultrasound which reveals a grossly enlarged right atrium, the septal leaflet of the tricuspid valve is displaced apically with a sail-like elongation.

3. A 29-year-old woman presents with her 4-week-old child who has had progressive cyanosis. She explains that today he appears blue in colour, she is also very concerned as he has been feeding poorly and appears to be breathing rapidly. She had an uneventful home delivery and has not attended routine antenatal care. On examination the child appears cyanosed and on auscultation of the praecordium you hear a harsh pansystolic murmur at the left lower sternal edge which is louder on expiration. You arrange a chest X-ray which reveals a boot-shaped heart.

4. A 29-year-old woman attends at 20 weeks' gestation and has so far had an uneventful pregnancy. You arrange for her 20-week fetal ultrasound which reveals a poorly developed left ventricle, a small left atrium, enlargement of the right side of the heart, a prominent pulmonary trunk and significant narrowing of the first part of the aorta.

5. A 68-year-old male presents with shortness of breath and postural hypotension. On examination you note that he has periorbital purpura, peripheral edema to the level of his knees, hepatomegaly and a pleural effusion on the left. Echocardiography reveals atrial thickening, bi-atrial enlargement, a sparkling appearance of the left ventricular myocardium and thickening of the left ventricular wall with decreased compliance.

See page 210 for answers.
See page 210 for answers.

ANSWERS

Chest pain 1

1. J. Pulmonary embolism
This is a condition in which a blood clot, usually from the lower limbs, travels to the lungs and occludes blood flow. A significant pulmonary embolism can lead to cardiac arrest.

2. E. Angina pectoris
Angina is by definition retrosternal chest pain or tightness which lasts for less than ten minutes in duration and is relieved by rest and is caused by myocardial ischaemia.

3. I. Pneumothorax
This patient has presented with a spontaneous pneumothorax. The chest pain is usually pleuritic in nature.

4. F. Oesophageal spasm
These are painful contractions within the muscular layer of the oesophagus, they can sometimes be precipitated by gastro-oesophageal reflux disease (GORD). Treatment initially involves drinking warm water, if this is unsuccessful sublingual nitrates can be used.

Chest pain 2

1. H. Pericarditis
Pericarditis is inflammation of the pericardium, a thin membrane that surrounds the heart. Viral infections are the most common cause of pericarditis.

2. C. Dissecting thoracic aortic aneurysm
Patients typically present with sudden onset chest pain with radiation to the back, classically described as "tearing" or "ripping". They may also present with shortness of breath and unilateral diminished or absent pulses.

3. K. Slipping rib syndrome
In this condition the cartilage in the lower ribs slips causing significant discomfort for the individual. There is usually a specific point of tenderness at the costal margin.

4. G. Myocardial infarction
This patient presents with the classic features for acute myocardial infarction, central chest pain lasting greater than ten minutes radiating to the left side and associated diaphoresis. He also has several risk factors for myocardial infarction. ECG changes in this case reflect those of an inferior ST elevation myocardial infarction.

Cardiac vessels

1. D. Left circumflex artery
This patient has had a lateral myocardial infarction.

2. C. Left anterior descending artery

This patient has had an anterior myocardial infarction.

3. H. Right coronary artery

This patient has had an inferior myocardial infarction.

Collapse 1

1. C. Diabetic neuropathy

This patient has poorly controlled diabetes as evidenced by repeated elevation of HbA1c measurements. This patient also has evidence of peripheral neuropathy and postural hypotension (a hallmark feature of diabetic autonomic neuropathy).

2. H. Pulmonary embolism

This is a condition in which a blood clot, usually from the legs, travels to the lungs and occludes blood flow. A significant pulmonary embolism can lead to cardiac arrest.

3. F. Hypoglycaemic episode

This patient has recently changed her diabetic medications and has not yet had breakfast. She has symptoms consistent with hypoglycaemia.

4. A. Addisonian crisis

This is a life-threatening condition which results in hypotension, hypoglycaemia and hyperkalaekmia. This patient requires urgent medical care.

Collapse 2

1. B. Cardiac tamponade

This occurs when the heart is compressed by fluid or gas within the pericardium. Metastatic cancer can cause malignant pericardial effusions resulting in cardiac tamponade.

2. G. Panic attack

These are brief episodes of intense anxiety in which patients may experience physical symptoms such as palpitations, shortness of breath and dizziness.

3. D. Epileptic seizure

This patient has had a tonic-clonic seizure; this type of seizure causes violent muscle contractions and loss of consciousness. This patient is also suffering from postictal symptoms.

4. E. Hypertrophic cardiomyopathy

The presentation and associated family history should raise suspicion about hypertrophic cardiomyopathy (HOCM). This patient has typical praecordial examination findings consistent with HOCM.

5. K. Vasovagal syncope

In this condition a patient collapses as a result of a reflex bradycardia and peripheral vasodilation because of exposure to a stressful trigger. In this case the most likely trigger is the vaccination.

Arrhythmias 1

1. **D. Cardiac tamponade**
   This occurs when the heart is compressed by fluid or gas within the pericardium. Electrical alternans is an ECG finding consistent with a large pericardial effusion and tamponade.

2. **Q. Wolff–Parkinson–White syndrome**
   In this condition an additional electrical pathway between the upper and lower chambers of the heart causes tachycardia. Typical ECG findings include short PR intervals and QRS complexes with associated slurred upstroke (delta waves).

3. **E. First-Degree heart block**
   The patient has an increased PR interval and is otherwise asymptomatic, he does not require any treatment for his presentation.

4. **B. Atrial Fibrillation**
   This patient has characteristic features of atrial fibrillation on her ECG, absent P waves and irregularly irregular QRS complexes.

5. **I. Right bundle branch block**
   This patient has the typical M shaped QRS complex (RSR' pattern) in leads V1-V3 and the W pattern in lead V6.

6. **K. Second-Degree heart block – Mobitz type 2**
   This patient presents with second degree AV block (Mobitz type 2). This presentation requires immediate hospital admission as this may result in haemodynamic compromise and progression to a third-degree heart block.

Arrhythmias 2

1. **A. Acute pericarditis**
   This condition results from inflammation of the pericardium. Typical exam findings include pleuritic chest pain and there may be an associated pericardial rub on auscultation. This patient has classic ECG findings: saddle shaped ST elevation in most limb leads with PR depression in most chest leads and reciprocal changes in aVR and V1.

2. **G. Hypertrophic cardiomyopathy**
   The presentation and associated family history should raise suspicion about hypertrophic cardiomyopathy. ECG findings in this case are typical of this condition.

3. **M. Third-Degree heart block**
   This patient has presented with a bradyarrhythmia and dissociation between the atrial and ventricular beats. This patient requires immediate hospital admission for cardiac pacing.

4. **L. Supraventricular tachycardia**
   This patient has presented with Supraventricular tachycardia (SVT), the best treatment options initially are non-pharmacological (Valsalva maneuver, carotid sinus massage).

5. H. Pulmonary embolism

This is a condition in which a blood clot, usually from the legs, travels to the lungs and blocks blood flow. Pulmonary embolism can lead to cardiac arrest. This patient has typical ECG findings including the classic $S_IQ_{III}T_{III}$ pattern.

Hypertension 1

1. E. Obstructive sleep apnoea

This condition causes multiple lapses in breathing during sleep. During sleep, patients experience upper airway collapse which results in snoring. Sleep apnoea can cause autonomic dysfunction which activates the sympathetic nervous system and results in hypertension.

2. H. Primary hyperaldosteronism

Also known as Conn's syndrome, this involves the over production of aldosterone by the adrenal glands which results in sodium retention and potassium excretion. Patients usually present with resistant hypertension and hypokalaemia (despite supplementation in this case).

3. I. Renal artery stenosis

This patient has uncontrolled hypertension despite the use of three agents, peripheral vascular disease, a history of flash pulmonary oedema and a bruit on abdominal examination. All of these features indicate renal artery stenosis as the most likely cause of her presentation.

4. C. Cushing syndrome

This patient has typical physical findings of Cushing syndrome. Failure to suppress cortisol levels following administration of low dose dexamethasone supports a diagnosis of Cushing syndrome.

Hypertension 2

1. B. Aortic coarctation

Coarctation of the aorta is narrowing of the aorta that reduces blood flow to the lower half of the body beyond this area. This condition is usually picked up during infancy, adults can present with it in later life with severe hypertension.

2. G. Polycystic kidney disease

This is an inherited condition in which cysts form within the kidneys, causing them to gradually enlarge and lose function. Hypertension and haematuria are common findings in this condition.

3. A. Acromegaly

This is a condition in adulthood in which excess growth hormone (GH) is produced by the pituitary gland. It causes overgrowth of the bones in the face, feet and hands. This condition can cause hypertension as it is associated with hyperinsulinemia, which stimulates reabsorption of sodium in the kidneys and sympathetic nervous system activity.

4. D. Hypothyroidism

This patient has classic physical features of hypothyroidism. Hypothyroidism can cause diastolic hypertension due to vascular endothelial dysfunction.

Murmurs 1

1. A. Aortic regurgitation

This condition occurs when the aortic valve does not close adequately, the result is retrograde flow of blood from the aorta into the left ventricle during systole. The murmur is best heard at Erb's point (the left sternal border at the level of the 3rd intercostal space). Clinical findings can include a water-hammer pulse (bounding pulse at the wrist), Corrigan's pulse (bounding pulse in the carotids), de Musset's sign (bobbing of the head in synchrony with the heart) and a wide pulse pressure.

2. C. Atrial myxoma

Myxomas are the most common primary cardiac neoplasm, they are most commonly found in the left atrium. The "tumor plop", which is a high-pitched sound usually heard in early diastole, occurs from either; 1) the mass on a stalk impacting against the myocardium, 2) tumour obstructing out flow or 3) tumour tensing.

3. E. Mitral regurgitation

This is when the mitral valve (between left atrium and left ventricle) is incompetent and blood flows from the left ventricle to the left atrium in retrograde manner during systole. With progressive regurgitation patients can develop shortness of breath especially on exertion and peripheral oedema. This patient has typical examination findings.

4. F. Mitral stenosis

This valve pathology is most commonly associated with rheumatic fever, usually in childhood. It presents with a diastolic murmur which is heard best at the 5th intercostal space on the mid-clavicular line. Following S2 (closure of the aortic valve) the opening snap of the stenotic mitral valve is heard followed by a low-pitched mid-diastolic murmur.

Murmurs 2

1. J. Tricuspid regurgitation

This patient presents with classical examination findings. Examination also typically reveals Carvallo's sign (murmur gets louder with deep inspiration), patients with severe tricuspid regurgitation may present with an accentuated jugular CV wave (Lancisi sign) and may also have congestive hepatopathy with a pulsatile liver.

2. I. Pulmonary regurgitation

This condition is most commonly found in association with pulmonary hypertension. This type of murmur is very similar to that seen with aortic regurgitation. The difference between the two being the location of where it is heard loudest; this murmur being heard loudest at the upper left sternal edge and that of aortic regurgitation being at the lower left sternal edge. A bounding pulse is also absent with pulmonary regurgitation.

3. H. Pericarditis

This condition results from inflammation of the pericardium. Typical exam findings include pleuritic chest pain and there may be an associated pericardial rub on auscultation. There is typically widespread ST segment changes on the ECG.

4. K. Tricuspid stenosis
This is narrowing of the tricuspid valve which blocks blood flow from the right atrium entering the right ventricle. This patient presents with classical clinical features of this condition.

CHA2DS2-VASc Scoring

1. E. CHA2DS2-VASc score 4
The correct answer is CHA2DS2-VASc score 4. He has scored one point for congestive cardiac failure, one point for hypertension and two points for age of 75 and above.

2. D. CHA2DS2-VASc score 3
The correct answer is CHA2DS2-VASc score 3. She has scored one point for hypertension, one point for age between 65 and 74 and one point for biological female sex.

3. B. CHA2DS2-VASc score 1
The correct answer is CHA2DS2-VASc score 1. He has scored one point for diabetes mellitus.

4. C. CHA2DS2-VASc score 2
The correct answer is CHA2DS2-VASc score 2. She has scored one point for vascular disease (peripheral arterial disease) and one point for biological female sex.

5. G. CHA2DS2-VASc score 6
The correct answer is CHA2DS2-VASc score 6. He has scored one point for hypertension, two points for age of 75 and above, two points for a history of thromboembolism and one point for biological female sex.

Hypertension grading

1. D. Grade 1 (mild) hypertension
Patients with a systolic BP of 140–159 mmHg and/or diastolic BP of 90–99 mmHg are classed as having grade 1 (mild) hypertension. See Australian heart foundation hypertension guidelines.

2. A. Optimal
Patients with a systolic BP of < 120 mmHg and diastolic BP of < 80 mmHg are classed as having an optimal blood pressure. See Australian heart foundation hypertension guidelines.

3. F. Grade 3 (severe) hypertension
Patients with a systolic BP of ≥ 180 mmHg and/or diastolic BP ≥ 110 mmHg are classed as having grade 3 (severe) hypertension. See Australian heart foundation hypertension guidelines.

4. G. Isolated systolic hypertension
Patients with a systolic BP > 140 mmHg and diastolic BP < 90 mmHg are classed as having isolated systolic hypertension. See Australian heart foundation hypertension guidelines.

5. B. Normal

Patients with a systolic BP of 120–129 mmHg and/or diastolic BP of 80–84 mmHg are classed as having a normal blood pressure. See Australian heart foundation hypertension guidelines.

Heart failure grading

1. D. NYHA Class IV

This patient reports that they are symptomatic at rest and with exertion, patients are graded from class I to class IV.

2. B. NYHA II

This patient is asymptomatic at rest, and becomes only mildly symptomatic with exertion, but is able to continue her normal activities of daily living. Patients are graded from class I to class IV.

3. C. NYHA III

This patient reports that they are asymptomatic at rest and have marked symptoms with exertion. Her symptoms are significantly impacting her daily activities. Patients are graded from class I to class IV.

Cardiac structure 1

1. A. Atrial septal defect

This is a congenital defect of the heart in which there is a persistence of communication in the septum between the atria of the heart. Most patients with a small atrial septal defect are asymptomatic.

2. M. Ventricular septal defect

This condition is commonly associated with Down syndrome. This patient has typical findings on auscultation.

3. I. Peripartum cardiomyopathy

This is weakness of the heart muscles which occur at the advance stages of pregnancy or after delivery. The heart becomes enlarged as a result and does not pump blood effectively resulting in heart failure.

4. C. Dilated cardiomyopathy

This is a condition which affects the muscles of the heart causing progressive dilatation and reduced capacity to pump effectively. It is likely that alcohol is the causative factor for this patient.

5. L. Transposition of the great arteries

This is a congenital cardiac defect in which the aorta is attached to the right ventricle of the heart rather than the left and the pulmonary artery is attached to the left ventricle of the heart rather than the right. Symptoms of this condition are usually present from birth.

Cardiac structure 2

1. G. Mitral valve prolapse

Also known as Barlow syndrome; this involves the bulging of one or both mitral valve leaflets into the left atrium during systole, allowing retrograde blood flow. The patient is typically asymptomatic.

2. D. Ebstein's anomaly

The use of lithium during the first trimester of pregnancy is associated with an increased risk of cardiac malformation. Apical displacement of the septal leaflet of the tricuspid valve by more than 8 mm/m2 with a sail-like elongation is diagnostic for Ebstein's anomaly.

3. K. Tetralogy of Fallot

This is a congenital heart condition involving four abnormalities (pulmonary stenosis, right ventricular hypertrophy, overriding aorta and ventricular septal defect, pneumonic PROV). A child with Tetralogy of Fallot usually has a harsh systolic crescendo decrescendo murmur at the left upper sternal margin which radiates through to the back (right ventricular outflow obstruction).

4. F. Hypoplastic left heart syndrome

This is a congenital heart condition which affects blood flow through the heart. In this condition the left side of the heart does not pump oxygenated blood through the body effectively as the left ventricle is too small.

5. J. Restrictive cardiomyopathy

This patient has a history and examination findings consistent with amyloidosis and echocardiograph findings support this. Amyloidosis is the most common cause of restrictive cardiomyopathy.

Respiratory

9

ARTERIAL BLOOD GAS INTERPRETATION 1

A. Metabolic acidosis – fully compensated
B. Metabolic acidosis – partial compensated
C. Metabolic acidosis – uncompensated
D. Metabolic alkalosis – fully compensated
E. Metabolic alkalosis – partial compensated
F. Metabolic alkalosis – uncompensated
G. Respiratory acidosis – fully compensated
H. Respiratory acidosis – partial compensated
 I. Respiratory acidosis – uncompensated
J. Respiratory alkalosis – fully compensated
K. Respiratory alkalosis – partial compensated
L. Respiratory alkalosis – uncompensated

For each of the following, what is the MOST likely diagnosis?

1. pH 7.32, $PaCO_2$ 36 mmHg and HCO_3 19 meq/L
2. pH 7.50, $PaCO_2$ 31 mmHg and HCO_3 24 meq/L
3. pH 7.49, $PaCO_2$ 41 mmHg and HCO_3 30 meq/L
4. pH 7.31, $PaCO_2$ 52 mmHg and HCO_3 27 meq/L

See page 234 for answers.

DOI: 10.1201/9781003459941-9

ARTERIAL BLOOD GAS INTERPRETATION 2

A. Metabolic acidosis – fully compensated
B. Metabolic acidosis – partial compensated
C. Metabolic acidosis – uncompensated
D. Metabolic alkalosis – fully compensated
E. Metabolic alkalosis – partial compensated
F. Metabolic alkalosis – uncompensated
G. Respiratory acidosis – fully compensated
H. Respiratory acidosis – partial compensated
I. Respiratory acidosis – uncompensated
J. Respiratory alkalosis – fully compensated
K. Respiratory alkalosis – partial compensated
L. Respiratory alkalosis – uncompensated

For each of the following, what is the MOST likely diagnosis?

1. pH 7.30, $PaCO_2$ 31mmHg and HCO_3 20 meq/L
2. pH 7.38, $PaCO_2$ 33 mmHg and HCO_3 21 meq/L
3. pH 7.36, $PaCO_2$ 54 mmHg and HCO_3 30 meq/L
4. pH 7.30, $PaCO_2$ 55 mmHg and HCO_3 23 meq/L

See page 234 for answers.

ENT 1

A. Acute mastoiditis
B. Acute otitis media
C. Acute rhinosinusitis
D. Allergic rhinitis
E. Bullous myringitis
F. Choanal atresia
G. Chronic otitis media
H. Chronic rhinosinusitis with polyps

I. Chronic rhinosinusitis without polyps
J. Deviated nasal septum
K. Granulomatosis with polyangiitis
L. Nasal foreign body
M. Otitis externa
N. Otitis media with effusion
O. Rhinitis medicamentosa

For each of the following, what is the MOST likely diagnosis?

1. A 14-year-old girl presents with a seven-week history of painless right ear discharge. The discharge is serous and without odour. She has a history of recurrent ear infections. On examination she has a temperature of 36.3°C and Weber test lateralises to the right side.

2. A 13-year-old boy presents with right sided ear pain and headache. His symptoms started two days ago and have progressively worsened. He now reports that he has swelling behind his right ear. On examination he has a temperature of 38.6°C, he has a bulging right tympanic membrane, there is swelling and pain on palpating posterior to his right ear.

3. A 21-year-old man presents to your clinic with epistaxis and nasal obstruction. He explains that his symptoms are associated with a cough, haemoptysis and pleuritic chest pain. Urine dipstick reveals haematuria and proteinuria. He has a strongly positive c-ANCA level detected in the serum.

4. You are working in a remote ED and are asked to review an 8-month-old child who has presented with a fever which started 24 hours ago. Her mother reports that she has been irritable and has been tugging on her left ear. On examination she has a temperature of 38.9°C, she also has an erythematous and bulging left tympanic membrane.

5. A 4-year-old girl presents to your clinic with a two-day history of foul-smelling brown discharge from her left nostril. Her mother explains that she has been complaining of a blocked nose for the past three days and today she has had an episode of epistaxis.

6. A 6-year-old boy presents to your clinic complaining of left ear pain and itch. He recently returned from Bali where his family took him for a vacation. He has been feeling unwell for the past two days, complaining of a sore throat and runny nose. He has no known sick contacts and his mother explains that he spent most of his time abroad playing with his siblings in the pool and on the beach. On examination there is narrowing of the ear canal and a large amount of exudate. He experiences significant pain when placing pressure on the tragus.

See pages 234–235 for answers.

ENT 2

A. Acute mastoiditis
B. Acute otitis media
C. Acute rhinosinusitis
D. Allergic rhinitis
E. Bullous myringitis
F. Choanal atresia
G. Chronic otitis media
H. Chronic rhinosinusitis with polyps
I. Chronic rhinosinusitis without polyps
J. Deviated nasal septum
K. Granulomatosis with polyangiitis
L. Nasal foreign body
M. Otitis externa
N. Otitis media with effusion
O. Rhinitis medicamentosa

For each of the following, what is the MOST likely diagnosis?

1. A 43-year-old male presents to your clinic with a three-month history of nasal congestion. He has been struggling to breathe through his nose and has had rhinorrhoea. He has a history of allergic rhinitis and has been using nasal decongestant sprays daily for the past four months. On examination his nasal mucous membranes appear beefy red in colour.

2. A 6-year-old boy attends your GP clinic with his mother who explains that she is concerned about his hearing. He has been turning the volume up to a high level on the television at home and has been getting into trouble at school with his teacher, who complains that he is not paying attention. He has been behaving this way for the past few weeks. On questioning he explains that his right ear feels blocked. He has a history of asthma and you note that he has presented several times with ear infections. On examination he is afebrile, the tympanic membrane on the right side is translucent with diminished mobility and an air fluid level is present behind it.

3. A 30-year-old man attends your GP clinic complaining of runny nose, with clear nasal discharge and watery eyes. He explains that his symptoms have been present for the past week and that they happen every year at roughly the same time. His symptoms are causing him difficulties with sleep and are affecting his function throughout the day.

4. A 37-year-old woman presents with right sided purulent nasal discharge for several weeks. You arrange for a CT scan which reveals vomer thickening, right sided narrowing of the posterior nasal passage and an airway width of 2 mm.

5. A 26-year-old man presents to your clinic with severe right sided ear pain and loss of hearing. On examination his right tympanic membrane is oedematous and covered in blood filled blisters.

6. A 21-year-old male presents to your clinic with a six-day history of thick green nasal discharge, left sided facial pain and a fever. He explains that his symptoms initially started with a sore throat and dry cough which resolved after two days, he improved slightly but his situation then began to deteriorate. On examination he has a temperature of 38.6°C, facial pain on percussion over the left cheek and pressure in the same location on leaning forward.

See pages 235–236 for answers.

PAEDIATRIC RESPIRATORY 1

A. Acute epiglottitis
B. Asthma
C. Bronchiolitis
D. Croup
E. Infectious mononucleosis
F. Influenza
G. Inhaled foreign body
H. Laryngitis
 I. Laryngomalacia
 J. Peritonsillar abscess
K. Pulmonary sequestration
L. Retropharyngeal abscess
M. Tonsillitis
N. Tracheo-Esophageal fistula
O. Upper airway cough syndrome

For each of the following, what is the MOST likely diagnosis?

1. A 6-week-old presents to your emergency department with her mother who is concerned about a fever. She has been coughing for the past four weeks particularly with feeding.

2. A 6-year-old boy presents to your GP clinic with a six-day history of cough. His mother explains that he has been coughing throughout the day due to irritation in the back of his throat. He describes this as if there is something "dripping down" the back of his throat. His mother further explains that he has also had a runny nose but denies any fever.

3. A 14-year-old girl attends your clinic complaining of a sore throat and dysphagia. She reports that this started one week ago and has progressively worsened and is associated with difficulty fully opening her mouth and some drooling. On

examination she is talking with a "hot potato" voice and she has deviation of her uvula to the right.

4. A 9-year-old boy presents to your clinic with a one-day history of myalgia and shortness of breath. His brother has similar symptoms which started two days ago. He has no medical history. On examination he has a temperature of 38.1°C, you note significant nasal discharge which is clear in colour, his chest is clear and he is talking in full sentences.

5. A 6-month-old girl attends your ED with her concerned mother. Her mother reports that her daughter had a two-day history of runny nose, cough and reduced feeds. She is also concerned that her daughter has been breathing rapidly throughout the day. On examination she has normal behaviour, a temperature of 37.3°C, respiratory rate of 56, saturations of 94% in room air, mild chest wall retraction and minimal wheeze bilaterally.

See page 236 for answers.

PAEDIATRIC RESPIRATORY 2

A. Acute epiglottitis
B. Asthma
C. Bronchiolitis
D. Croup
E. Infectious mononucleosis
F. Influenza
G. Inhaled foreign body
H. Laryngitis
 I. Laryngomalacia
 J. Peritonsillar abscess
K. Pulmonary sequestration
L. Retropharyngeal abscess
M. Tonsillitis
N. Tracheo-Esophageal fistula
O. Upper airway cough syndrome

For each of the following, what is the MOST likely diagnosis?

1. A 4-year-old boy presents to your emergency department with a five-day history of fever and reduced oral intake. On examination he appears unwell, has a temperature of 39.2°C, is drooling and seated leaning forward with his neck extended.

2. A 4-year-old girl attends your clinic with her mother. For the past three days she has been coughing intermittently and has a low-grade fever. In clinic you

observe a barking cough, she has intermittent inspiratory stridor at rest and moderate chest wall retractions. Her chest is otherwise clear.

3. A 13-year-old girl presents to your emergency department with a sore throat, odynophagia and fever. She explains that her symptoms initially started a week ago and have progressively worsened. On examination she is talking with a "hot potato" voice, has a temperature of 40.2°C, has some stiffness in her neck and pain on palpation of her anterior neck. A lateral X-ray of her neck reveals widening of the prevertebral soft tissue and swelling posterior to the pharynx.

4. A 16-year-old boy presents to your GP clinic complaining of a two-day history of sore throat and fever. He has no significant medical history and takes no regular medication. On examination he has a temperature of 37.9°C, he has enlarged tonsils covered in a white film, cervical lymph nodes are enlarged and he has splenomegaly. A heterophile antibody test returns a positive result.

5. A 16-year-old girl presents with a one-day history of sore throat. She has been maintaining fluids but struggles to swallow food. On examination she has swelling of bilateral tonsils which are erythematous and covered with white exudate bilaterally, she has a temperature of 38.8°C. Abdominal examination is unremarkable.

See pages 236–237 for answers.

PAEDIATRIC RESPIRATORY 3

A. Acute epiglottitis
B. Asthma
C. Bronchiolitis
D. Croup
E. Infectious mononucleosis
F. Influenza
G. Inhaled foreign body
H. Laryngitis
I. Laryngomalacia
J. Peritonsillar abscess
K. Pulmonary sequestration
L. Retropharyngeal abscess
M. Tonsillitis
N. Tracheo-Esophageal fistula
O. Upper airway cough syndrome

For each of the following, what is the MOST likely diagnosis?

1. A 20-month-old boy is brought to your ED by ambulance with a complaint of acute respiratory distress. His father is in attendance and explains that he has been well and was playing with his older sister just before his symptoms started. On examination he has a temperature of 37.9°C, marked stridor, saturations of 91% at room air and a clear chest.

2. A 6-year-old boy presents to your clinic with a history of recurrent chest infections affecting the left lower lobe of his lungs. CT angiography reveals anomalous blood supply to the affected lobe from the descending thoracic aorta.

3. A 6-week-old child is brought to your clinic by her mother, who is concerned about noisy breathing she has noticed for the past five weeks. Her mother explains that the noise is more noticeable when she lays her flat or when she is sleeping, it disappears when she changes her position.

4. An 8-year-old girl presents to your clinic with her father, she has been coughing for the past two weeks. Her cough is non-productive, it is associated with chest tightness and wheeze. She explains that her symptoms are worse at night and first thing in the morning when she wakes, she has had broken sleep over this period. She has not had a fever.

5. A 15-year-old girl presents to your clinic complaining of a sore throat and dysphagia. Her symptoms have been present for the past seven days and she has developed a hoarse voice since yesterday. On examination she has erythema at the back of her throat, cervical lymphadenopathy and a temperature of 37.6°C.

See page 237 for answers.

RESPIRATORY CONDITIONS 1

A. **Acute pulmonary oedema**
B. **Asthma**
C. **Bronchiectasis**
D. **Chronic obstructive airways disease**
E. **Churg–Strauss syndrome**
F. **Cystic fibrosis**
G. **Empyema**
H. **Goodpasture syndrome**
I. **Granulomatosis with polyangiitis**
J. **Haemothorax**
K. **Idiopathic pulmonary fibrosis**
L. **Lobar pneumonia**
M. **Lung abscess**
N. **Lung cancer**

O. Mesothelioma
P. Mycoplasma pneumonia
Q. Pneumothorax
R. Pulmonary aspergillosis
S. Pulmonary embolism
T. Sarcoidosis
U. Silicosis
V. Tuberculosis

For each of the following, what is the MOST likely diagnosis?

1. A 40-year-old Caucasian woman presents with a four-month history of dry cough and associated shortness of breath. She reports that she has been significantly fatigued during this period of time and has lost 3 kg. On examination she has a bluish-red rash over her nose, her chest sounds clear. Chest X-ray reveals bilateral hilar lymphadenopathy.

2. A 32-year-old woman presents to your clinic with a history of cough. She explains that her symptoms are fever, haemoptysis and shortness of breath. She was previously started on broad spectrum antibiotics but has had no response to these. She has breast cancer and is currently undergoing chemotherapy. You arrange for a CT chest which reveals a halo sign.

3. A 28-year-old receptionist presents to your clinic complaining of a long history of nocturnal cough which has been waking her nightly for the past month, she explains that she has had these symptoms in the past but they have become considerably more bothersome. She explains that she also has chest tightness and wheeze throughout the day on most days during this period.

4. An 18-year-old basketball player is brought into your emergency department with sudden onset shortness of breath associated with right sided chest pain. He appears pale in colour and is struggling to talk. On examination he has a temperature of 36.7°C and saturations of 91% at room air, he has decreased breath sound on the right side of his chest and associated tracheal deviation towards the left.

5. A 32-year-old male presents with a two-week history of cough and haemoptysis. He has no associated symptoms. On examination he has a blood pressure of 158/94 mmHg, temperature of 36.6°C, heart rate of 92 beats per minute and a respiratory rate of 24 breaths per minute. He has bilateral crackles in his lungs and peripheral oedema. Dipstick reveals haematuria. You send the urine off which reveals the presence of red cell casts. A biopsy is arranged which shows strongly positive linear staining of glomerular capillaries for IgG.

6. A 68-year-old male presents to your emergency department with a two-week history of productive cough and fever. He also reports left sided pleuritic chest pain. On examination he has a temperature of 39.1°C, heart rate of 112 beats per minute and a respiratory rate of 24 breaths per minute. He is also found to have reduced breath sounds in the lower half of the left chest. A CT of the chest is requested, split pleura sign on the left side is observed.

See pages 237–238 for answers.

RESPIRATORY CONDITIONS 2

A. Acute pulmonary oedema
B. Asthma
C. Bronchiectasis
D. Chronic obstructive airways disease
E. Churg–Strauss syndrome
F. Cystic fibrosis
G. Empyema
H. Goodpasture syndrome
 I. Granulomatosis with polyangiitis
J. Haemothorax
K. Idiopathic pulmonary fibrosis
L. Lobar pneumonia
M. Lung abscess
N. Lung cancer
O. Mesothelioma
P. Mycoplasma pneumonia
Q. Pneumothorax
R. Pulmonary aspergillosis
S. Pulmonary embolism
T. Sarcoidosis
U. Silicosis
V. Tuberculosis

For each of the following, what is the MOST likely diagnosis?

1. A 33-year-old sandblaster presents to your GP clinic for the first time with a 12-month history of productive cough and shortness of breath on exertion. He has had multiple courses of antibiotics during this period of time which have had little effect. His chest X-ray reveals bilateral hilar adenopathy with egg shell calcification.

2. A 61-year-old man presents to your clinic with a five-day history of fever associated with a productive cough. He reports that his symptoms have worsened and his sputum is now rust coloured. On examination he has a temperature of 38.5°C, heart rate of 106 beats per minute and a respiratory rate of 22 breaths per minute. There are bronchial breath sounds and dullness to percussion in the left lower zone.

3. A 12-year-old refugee attends your clinic as he has been suffering from a chronic upper respiratory tract infection for the past six weeks. He has had a course of amoxicillin without any response to treatment. He explains that he has had a cough and runny nose intermittently for the past two years. He also reports that he snores at night. He further explains that he has had very thick

and greasy white stools during this period. He denies any shortness of breath or haemoptysis. He has had all of his catch-up immunisations.

4. A 58-year-old labourer presents to your consulting rooms complaining of a two-month history of dry cough which is now associated with haemoptysis. He is a non-smoker and reports that he has lost 6 kg over this period of time.

5. A 66-year-old man presents to your emergency department with a two-week history of cough and fever. He was recently admitted to the hospital for a stroke but has no other significant medical history. He previously smoked a pack of cigarettes a day but quit smoking 15 years ago. On examination he has a temperature of 38.8°C, heart rate of 110 beats per minute and a respiratory rate of 26 breaths per minute. A chest X-ray is performed which reveals a round shaped cavity containing an air-fluid level in the right middle lobe.

See page 238 for answers.

RESPIRATORY CONDITIONS 3

A. Acute pulmonary oedema
B. Asthma
C. Bronchiectasis
D. Chronic obstructive airways disease
E. Churg–Strauss syndrome
F. Cystic fibrosis
G. Empyema
H. Goodpasture syndrome
I. Granulomatosis with polyangiitis
J. Haemothorax
K. Idiopathic pulmonary fibrosis
L. Lobar pneumonia
M. Lung abscess
N. Lung cancer
O. Mesothelioma
P. Mycoplasma pneumonia
Q. Pneumothorax
R. Pulmonary aspergillosis
S. Pulmonary embolism
T. Sarcoidosis
U. Silicosis
V. Tuberculosis

For each of the following, what is the MOST likely diagnosis?

1. A 32-year-old receptionist attends your clinic with a history of sudden onset shortness of breath and pleuritic chest pain. She reports that she has also developed a non-productive cough. Last week she had a LLETZ procedure following the discovery of abnormal cervical cell changes detected on her recent cervical screening test. She is also a smoker.

2. A 42-year-old refugee presents at your clinic complaining of a three-month history of cough with haemoptysis, he also reports pleuritic chest pain. He weighs 58 kg; he tells you that he last weighed himself shortly before his symptoms commenced and he was 66 kg. On examination he has a temperature of 37.7°C. You perform a chest X-ray which reveals patchy airway opacities in the left upper lobe with a cavitary lesion.

3. A 61-year-old woman attends your GP clinic. She reports a one-year history of chronic cough, which is worse in the morning and is associated with thick, foul smelling sputum production. You review her file and note that she has been prescribed antibiotics on several occasions by other GPs at your clinic for similar such presentations. She reports that she has recently noticed that her sputum has become blood tinged. Her chest X-ray reveals tram tracking at the bases of her lungs. She is a non-smoker.

4. A 26-year-old woman presents to your clinic with epistaxis and nasal obstruction. She explains that her symptoms are associated with a cough, haemoptysis and pleuritic chest pain. Urine dipstick reveals haematuria and proteinuria. She has a strongly positive c-ANCA level detected in the serum.

5. A 25-year-old woman is brought into your emergency department after a motor bike accident. She is struggling to breath on review and loses consciousness. On examination she has a BP of 82/60 mmHg, heart rate of 120 beats per minute and respiratory rate of 30 breaths per minute. She has bruising down the right side of her chest wall, her trachea is deviated to the left, she has absent breath sounds on the right side and there is dullness to percussion on this side also.

See pages 238–239 for answers.

RESPIRATORY CONDITIONS 4

A. Acute pulmonary oedema
B. Asthma
C. Bronchiectasis
D. Chronic obstructive airways disease
E. Churg–Strauss syndrome
F. Cystic fibrosis

G. **Empyema**

H. **Goodpasture syndrome**

I. **Granulomatosis with polyangiitis**

J. **Haemothorax**

K. **Idiopathic pulmonary fibrosis**

L. **Lobar pneumonia**

M. **Lung abscess**

N. **Lung cancer**

O. **Mesothelioma**

P. **Mycoplasma pneumonia**

Q. **Pneumothorax**

R. **Pulmonary aspergillosis**

S. **Pulmonary embolism**

T. **Sarcoidosis**

U. **Silicosis**

V. **Tuberculosis**

For each of the following, what is the MOST likely diagnosis?

1. A 63-year-old retired fire fighter presents to see you regarding shortness of breath on exertion and associated loss of weight. You perform a chest X-ray which reveals a small right sided pleural effusion and right sided pleural thickening.

2. A 66-year-old man presents with shortness of breath. He explains that his symptoms have been present for the past 12 months and are progressively worsening, they are worse with exertion and are associated with a dry cough. He previously smoked a packet of cigarettes a day but quit 20 years ago. On examination his has fine bibasal crackles, clubbing of his fingers, a JVP of 3 cm and no evidence of peripheral oedema. Spirometry is performed which reveals FEV1 1.59 L (51% of predicted), FVC 1.68 L (40% of predicted) and FEV1/FVC 94.6%.

3. A 37-year-old woman presents with worsening cough. She reports that recently she has had episodes of haemoptysis. She is a non-smoker, has a history of asthma and hay fever. On examination she has diffuse high pitched expiratory rhonchi and wheeze bilaterally. You arrange for laboratory investigations which reveal eosinophilia and positive p-ANCA.

4. A 53-year-old ex-smoker attends your clinic for review, he reports that over the past six months he has been increasingly short of breath on moderate levels of exertion. He has smoked a pack of cigarettes daily since the age of 19. On examination he has a barrel chest, faint wheeze throughout his chest and Hoover's sign is present. A chest X-ray is requested which demonstrates hyperinflation. You perform a spirometry which reveals an FEV1/FVC of 0.67 and an FEV1 of 74% predicted.

5. A 68-year-old man presents to your emergency department with shortness of breath associated with coughing. He has been symptomatic for the past six days and has progressively worsened. He reports that he has become increasingly fatigued and struggles with his daily activities. He has a history of T2DM,

hypertension and hyperlipidaemia. On examination he is afebrile, has a JVP of 6 cm, his chest has bilateral basal crackles and he has bilateral pitting oedema to the level of his knees.

See page 239 for answers.

PNEUMOTHORAX

A. **Catamenial pneumothorax**
B. **Chylothorax**
C. **Fibrothorax**
D. **Haemothorax**
E. **Haemopneumothorax**
F. **Hydropneumothorax**
G. **Primary spontaneous pneumothorax**
H. **Secondary spontaneous pneumothorax**
I. **Tension pneumothorax**

For each of the following, what is the MOST likely diagnosis?

1. An 18-year-old netball player is brought into your emergency department via ambulance with sudden onset shortness of breath associated with right sided chest pain. The ambulance officer explains that she was playing at a local tournament and took a hard hit from another player while trying to obtain the ball, she fell onto her right side and became extremely short of breath. She was able to explain to the arriving ambulance officers what had occurred but had begun to deteriorate rapidly shortly after. On arrival she is pale in colour and is struggling to talk. On examination she has a temperature of 36.9°C, respiratory rate of 36, heart rate of 124, blood pressure of 88/62 mmHg and saturations of 89% at room air, she has decreased breath sounds on the right side of her chest and associated tracheal deviation towards the left. She is a non-smoker, has no significant past medical history and does not use any regular medication other than the oral contraceptive pill.

2. You are a house officer with the surgical unit and are called to the ward to see a 68-year-old male who is complaining of shortness of breath. His symptoms have progressively worsened over the past two days since he had an oesophagectomy. He has a history of oesophageal cancer, hypertension and T2DM. On examination there is dullness to percussion and absent breath sounds on the right side. He is afebrile and has significant cervical lymphadenopathy on palpation of the anterior neck. A chest X-ray is performed which reveals a right sided pleural effusion. Thoracocentesis is performed and 500 ml of milky fluid is removed.

3. A 62-year-old ex-smoker is brought into your rural emergency department with acute onset of shortness of breath and left sided chest pain. The patient appears to be distressed and is struggling to talk, his partner explains that he had gotten up to use the bathroom and on his return his symptoms came on suddenly, she subsequently called for an ambulance. On examination he is pale and obviously distressed, he has a temperature of 36.3°C and saturations of 90% at room air, he has decreased breath sounds on the left side of his chest with associated hyperresonance and the trachea is midline. He has some paperwork from his GP and a recent spirometry reading from six months ago which confirms a diagnosis of COPD. He has had his influenza vaccination this year and has not had a chest infection in over 12 months.

4. A 36-year-old woman presents to your emergency department with chest pain and shortness of breath. She reports that she has had similar episodes every month for the past six months and has been admitted on three occasions during this time for spontaneous pneumothoraces. She suffers from endometriosis and her period started two days ago. You arrange for a chest X-ray which reveals a right sided pneumothorax.

5. A 21-year-old fit and healthy male is brought into your emergency department with shortness of breath associated with right sided chest pain, he explains that his symptoms started two days ago and have not improved. He is pale in colour and is talking in full sentences. On examination he has a temperature of 36.7°C, BP of 124/86 mmHg, RR of 18 and saturations of 98% at room air, he has markedly decreased breath sounds on the right side of his chest, accessory muscle use and the trachea is midline. He is a non-smoker, has no significant past medical history and does not use any regular medication. His mother reports that he was seated on a chair just prior to onset of his symptoms.

See pages 239–240 for answers.

OCCUPATIONAL RESPIRATORY CONDITIONS 1

A. **Asbestosis**
B. **Bronchiolitis obliterans**
C. **Brucellosis**
D. **Byssinosis**
E. **Coal workers pneumoconiosis**
F. **Hypersensitivity pneumonitis**
G. **Legionnaires' disease**
H. **Occupational asthma**
I. **Psittacosis**
J. **Q fever**
K. **Silicosis**

For each of the following, what is the MOST likely diagnosis?

1. A 42-year-old woman presents with right sided chest pain and cough that has persisted for the past three weeks. She was seen by another GP and commenced on a course of amoxicillin last week without any resolution of her symptoms. She lives at home alone and keeps many pigeons which she races competitively on a monthly basis. On examination she appears to be comfortable, has a temperature of 37.0°C, regular HR of 64, RR of 20 and saturations of 95% at room air. Her chest has diffuse expiratory crackles bilaterally. She has not had any sick contacts nor has she travelled recently.

2. A 32-year-old male presents with a four-year history of cough. He reports that during this time he has also been suffering from episodes of shortness of breath, wheeze and chest tightness. He is a vehicle body spray painter and uses mostly isocyanate-based aerosol paints. He reports that his symptoms are worse whilst at work.

3. A 53-year-old fire fighter presents to your clinic with worsening shortness of breath. He has no significant medical history, takes no regular medication and has no history of cigarette smoking. On examination you note fine crackles in bilateral lower zones. A chest X-ray is arranged which reveals irregular opacities associated with a fine reticular pattern and multiple pleural plaques.

4. A 36-year-old man presents with a 12-month history of progressive shortness of breath. He reports that his symptoms are worse with exertion and are associated with a dry cough. He is a non-smoker, has no medical history of note and has been working as a coal mine engineer for the past 11 years. On examination his chest is clear. A chest X-ray reveals small irregular opacities throughout the chest measuring between 1–5 mm.

5. A 27-year-old factory worker presents to your clinic with a two-year history of cough and worsening shortness of breath. He has no medical history of note and is a non-smoker. He works at a popcorn manufacturing company and has done so for the past three years. HRCT shows bronchial wall thickening and mosaic attenuation with air trapping.

See page 240 for answers.

OCCUPATIONAL RESPIRATORY CONDITIONS 2

A. Asbestosis
B. Bronchiolitis obliterans
C. Brucellosis
D. Byssinosis
E. Coal workers pneumoconiosis
F. Hypersensitivity pneumonitis
G. Legionnaires' disease

H. Occupational asthma
I. Psittacosis
J. Q fever
K. Silicosis

For each of the following, what is the MOST likely diagnosis?

1. A 53-year-old farmer presents to your GP clinic complaining of worsening shortness of breath on exertion over the past eight days. He reports that he gets chest tightness during the episodes, he also suffers from tightness in his chest. He further reports that he has had intermittent fevers over the past four days. He tells you that his symptoms are usually worse when he is on the farm. He has no significant medical history, takes no regular medications and has never smoked cigarettes.

2. A 38-year-old cotton factory worker presents with a 12-month history of persistent dry cough. He explains that his cough has gradually worsened and is associated with a small amount of sputum production. He is a non-smoker and has no significant medical history.

3. A 45-year-old man presents with a six-month history of productive cough and shortness of breath on exertion. He is a non-smoker and has no significant medical history. He has worked as a sand blaster for 20 years and reports no significant family medical history. He has seen several doctors who have prescribed him a variety of antibiotics and steroids to no avail. A chest X-ray reveals bilateral hilar adenopathy with egg shell calcification.

4. A 58-year-old man presents to your emergency department with worsening shortness of breath. He has had a four-day history of cough productive of thick yellow sputum, myalgia and fever. He is an air conditioner repairman and works in high rise buildings. He has a history of type 2 diabetes mellitus and has been smoking a packet of cigarettes a day for the past 30 years. He is compliant with his medications. On examination he has a temperature of 38.0°C, regular HR of 104, RR of 26 and saturations of 93% at room air. His chest has diffuse expiratory crackles bilaterally. He has not had any sick contacts nor has he travelled recently.

5. A 26-year-old man presents to your clinic with a low-grade fever and cough. He also reports myalgia and joint pain. His symptoms have been present for the past two days and are worsening. He has no significant medical history. He has recently returned from travel to Portugal, three days ago, where he worked at a dairy farm for a year. He explains that he is normally fit and active, he also explains that he eats healthy and has been consuming unpasteurised dairy products while abroad.

See pages 240–241 for answers.

LUNG CANCER

A. **Bronchial carcinoid**
B. **Bronchioloalveolar carcinoma**
C. **Large cell lung carcinoma**
D. **Lung adenocarcinoma**
E. **Lymphoma**
 F. **Mesothelioma**
G. **Pancoast tumor**
H. **Small cell lung carcinoma**
 I. **Squamous cell lung cancer**
 J. **Teratoma**

For each of the following, what is the MOST likely diagnosis?

1. A 50-year-old accountant presents with a nine-month history of cough. He has no significant medical history and he is a non-smoker. A chest X-ray reveals an irregularly shaped lesion in the left lung. Bronchoscopy is normal.
2. A 70-year-old woman presents to your clinic with a three-month history of right shoulder pain radiating into her scapula and axilla. She reports that she has also had progressive weakness in her right upper limb particularly in her hand. She has not had any trauma. On examination she has reduced grip strength in her right hand.
3. A 46-year-old man presents with a chronic cough. His symptoms have been present for 12 months and have recently been associated with haemoptysis and dyspnoea. He has no significant medical history and is a non-smoker. You arrange for bronchoscopy which reveals a cherry red lesion in the left superior lobar bronchus.
4. A 67-year-old man presents with an exacerbation of COPD, he has had multiple similar episodes this year. You have not been able to successfully treat his current symptoms with the use of oral steroids and antibiotics and have arranged for a chest X-ray which reveals a 2 cm mass in the left lower lobe. Blood electrolyte levels reveal hyponatraemia.
5. A 60-year-old retired pipe lagger presents to see you regarding shortness of breath on exertion and associated loss of weight. You perform a chest X-ray which reveals a small right sided pleural effusion and right sided pleural thickening.

See page 241 for answers.

CHEST IMAGING FINDINGS 1

A. Acute pulmonary edema
B. Asbestosis
C. Bronchiectasis
D. Chronic obstructive airways disease
E. Coarctation of the aorta
F. Left atrial enlargement
G. Lobar consolidation
H. Lung abscess
I. Pericardial effusion
J. Pleural effusion
K. Pleural empyema
L. Pneumomediastinum
M. Pneumothorax
N. Pulmonary embolism
O. Round atelectasis
P. Sarcoidosis
Q. Tetralogy of Fallot
R. Total anomalous pulmonary venous return
S. Transposition of the great arteries

For each of the following, what is the MOST likely diagnosis?

1. Double density sign seen on a chest X-ray.
2. Blunting of the costophrenic angle seen on a chest X-ray.
3. Double diaphragm sign seen on a supine chest X-ray.
4. Split pleura sign seen on CT of the chest.
5. Cluster of black pearls sign seen on contrast enhanced CT of the chest.
6. Holly leaf sign seen on a chest X-ray.
7. Bulging fissure sign on chest X-ray.

See pages 241–242 for answers.

See pages 241–242 for answers.

CHEST IMAGING FINDINGS 2

A. Acute pulmonary edema
B. Asbestosis
C. Bronchiectasis
D. Chronic obstructive airways disease
E. Coarctation of the aorta

F. Left atrial enlargement
G. Lobar consolidation
H. Lung abscess
 I. Pericardial effusion
 J. Pleural effusion
K. Pleural empyema
L. Pneumomediastinum
M. Pneumothorax
N. Pulmonary embolism
O. Round atelectasis
 P. Sarcoidosis
Q. Tetralogy of Fallot
R. Total anomalous pulmonary venous return
S. Transposition of the great arteries

For each of the following, what is the MOST likely diagnosis?

1. Water bottle sign seen on a chest X-ray.
2. Batwing appearance of chest X-ray.
3. Comet tail sign seen on CT of the chest.
4. Boot shaped heart seen on chest X-ray.
5. Egg on a string sign seen on chest X-ray.
6. Signet ring sign seen on CT of chest.

See page 242 for answers.

CHEST IMAGING FINDINGS 3

A. Acute pulmonary edema
B. Asbestosis
C. Bronchiectasis
D. Chronic obstructive airways disease
E. Coarctation of the aorta
 F. Left atrial enlargement
G. Lobar consolidation
H. Lung abscess
 I. Pericardial effusion
 J. Pleural effusion
K. Pleural empyema
L. Pneumomediastinum
M. Pneumothorax
N. Pulmonary embolism
O. Round atelectasis

P. Sarcoidosis
Q. Tetralogy of Fallot
R. Total anomalous pulmonary venous return
S. Transposition of the great arteries

For each of the following, what is the MOST likely diagnosis?

1. Figure 3 sign seen on a chest X-ray.
2. Snowman sign seen on chest X-ray.
3. Sabre-sheath trachea seen on CT of the chest.
4. Continuous diaphragm sign seen on chest X-ray.
5. Fleischner sign seen on chest X-ray.
6. Irregularly shaped cavity with an air fluid level seen on a chest X-ray.

See pages 242–243 for answers.

RESPIRATORY MICROBIOLOGY 1

A. Aspergillus fumigatus
B. Bordetella pertussis
C. Chlamydia psittaci
D. Haemophilus influenzae
E. Legionella pneumophila
F. Mycoplasma pneumoniae
G. Mycoplasma tuberculosis
H. Pneumocystis jirovecii
 I. Pseudomonas aeruginosa
J. Staphylococcus aureus
K. Streptococcus pneumoniae
L. Streptococcus pyogenes

For each of the following situations, what is the MOST likely cause?

1. A 58-year-old man presents with worsening shortness of breath. He has had a
   four-day history of cough productive of thick yellow sputum, myalgia and fever.
   He is an air conditioner repairman and works in high-rise buildings. He has a
   history of type 2 diabetes mellitus and has been smoking a packet of cigarettes a
   day for the past 30 years. He is compliant with his medications. On examination
   he has a temperature of 38.0°C, regular HR of 104, RR of 26 and saturations of
   93% at room air. His chest has diffuse expiratory crackles bilaterally. He has
   not had any sick contacts nor has he travelled recently.
2. A 45-year-old presents with a two-week history of cough and associated shortness of breath. He has a history of hypertension, appendicectomy at the age of

12 and recent HIV diagnosis. He has recently been commenced on anti-retroviral medications. Chest examination is unremarkable and a chest X-ray reveals bilateral diffuse alveolo-interstitial infiltration.

3. A 3-year-old boy attends your emergency department with his mother who is concerned about a rash which has developed today. The rash covers his entire body except for his palms, soles of his feet and his face. His mother explains that he has had a fever for the past two days and a sore throat. On examination he has white coloured discharge covering the back of his throat, a generalised erythematous rash that has a texture like sandpaper, he also has cervical and submandibular lymphadenopathy.

4. A 38-year-old IV drug user attends your emergency department with a two-day history of fever, productive cough and shortness of breath. On examination he has a temperature of 38.6°C, a respiratory rate of 24 breaths per minute and a heart rate of 117 beats per minute. A chest X-ray is arranged which reveals multiple round shaped cavities containing air fluid levels in bilateral lungs.

5. A 59-year-old woman presents with a 12-month history of cough, particularly in the morning. Her cough is associated with production of thick, foul-smelling sputum. She has had several courses of antibiotics to help her treat her symptoms but has had no success with treatment. She has no significant history of note and is a non-smoker. Chest X-ray shows tram tracking at the bases of bilateral lungs. You arrange for a sputum MCS.

See page 243 for answers.

RESPIRATORY MICROBIOLOGY 2

A. **Aspergillus fumigatus**
B. **Bordetella pertussis**
C. **Chlamydia psittaci**
D. **Haemophilus influenzae**
E. **Legionella pneumophila**
F. **Mycoplasma pneumoniae**
G. **Mycoplasma tuberculosis**
H. **Pneumocystis jirovecii**
I. **Pseudomonas aeruginosa**
J. **Staphylococcus aureus**
K. **Streptococcus pneumoniae**
L. **Streptococcus pyogenes**

For each of the following situations, what is the MOST likely cause?

1. A 65-year-old man presents to your clinic with a four-day history of fever and productive cough. He explains that his symptoms have worsened and he now has rust coloured sputum. He has had no recent illness and has no significant medical history of note. On examination he has a temperature of 38.7°C, heart rate of 110 beats per minute and a respiratory rate of 24 breaths per minute. There are bronchial breath sounds and dullness to percussion in the right lower zone.

2. A 36-year-old woman presents with a one-week history of productive cough. She explains to you that her symptoms are associated with a low-grade fever, sore throat and muscle pain. The cough is productive of white coloured sputum. On examination she has a temperature of 37.8°C and bilateral crackles in mid and lower zones.

3. A 15-year-old girl presents to your emergency with fever associated with short-ness of breath. She has a history of recurrent chest infections secondary to cys-tic fibrosis. On examination he has a temperature of 38.5°C, a respiratory rate of 26 breaths per minute, saturations of 90% at room air and a heart rate of 122 beats per minute.

4. A 38-year-old man presents with a 12-day history of chest pain. His symptoms are associated with fever, diaphoresis and myalgia. He was seen in the local emergency department a week ago and commenced on amoxicillin but this did not help his symptoms. He is a farm worker and has many parakeets he cares for at home, he has no significant medical history of note. On examination he appears to be comfortable, has a temperature of 37.2°C, regular heart rate of 76, respiratory rate of 18 and saturations of 96% at room air. On auscultation he has diffuse expiratory crackles bilaterally.

5. A 4-year-old child is brought into your emergency department as he has been having bouts of coughing which end in vomiting. His mother is very distressed as a result of his presentation. He has no significant medical history; he has not been vaccinated as his mother is opposed to vaccinations.

6. A 26-year-old refugee presents with a two-day history of fever, sweats and productive cough with haemoptysis. On examination he has a temperature of 37.9°C. You perform a chest X-ray which reveals patchy airway opacities in the left upper lobe with a cavitary lesion. Ziehl–Neelsen stain is performed and positive for acid fast bacilli.

See pages 243–244 for answers.

ANSWERS

Arterial blood gas interpretation 1

1. C. Metabolic acidosis – uncompensated

Normal ranges for blood gases are: pH between 7.35–7.45, $PaCO_2$ between 35–45 mmHg and HCO_3 is 22–26 meq/L. In uncompensated metabolic acidosis pH is reduced, $PaCO_2$ is normal and HCO_3 is reduced.

2. L. Respiratory alkalosis – uncompensated

Normal ranges for blood gases are: pH between 7.35–7.45, $PaCO_2$ between 35–45 mmHg and HCO_3 is 22–26 meq/L. In uncompensated respiratory alkalosis pH is elevated, $PaCO_2$ is decreased and HCO_3 is normal.

3. E. Metabolic alkalosis – partially compensated

Normal ranges for blood gases are: pH between 7.35–7.45, $PaCO_2$ between 35–45 mmHg and HCO_3 is 22–26 meq/L. In partially compensated metabolic alkalosis pH is elevated, $PaCO_2$ is elevated and HCO_3 is elevated.

*4. H. Respiratory acidosis – partially compensated

Normal ranges for blood gases are: pH between 7.35–7.45, $PaCO_2$ between 35–45 mmHg and HCO_3 is 22–26 meq/L. In partially compensated respiratory acidosis pH is reduced, $PaCO_2$ is elevated and HCO_3 is elevated.

Arterial blood gas interpretation 2

1. B. Metabolic acidosis – partially compensated

Normal ranges for blood gases are: pH between 7.35–7.45, $PaCO_2$ between 35–45 mmHg and HCO_3 is 22–26 meq/L. In partially compensated metabolic acidosis pH is reduced, $PaCO_2$ is reduced and HCO_3 is reduced.

2. J. Respiratory alkalosis – fully compensated

Normal ranges for blood gases are: pH between 7.35–7.45, $PaCO_2$ between 35–45 mmHg and HCO_3 is 22–26 meq/L. In fully compensated respiratory alkalosis pH is normal, $PaCO_2$ is decreased and HCO_3 is decreased.

3. G. Respiratory acidosis – fully compensated

Normal ranges for blood gases are: pH between 7.35–7.45, $PaCO_2$ between 35–45 mmHg and HCO_3 is 22–26 meq/L. In fully compensated respiratory acidosis pH is normal, $PaCO_2$ is elevated and HCO_3 is elevated.

4. I. Respiratory acidosis – uncompensated

Normal ranges for blood gases are: pH between 7.35–7.45, $PaCO_2$ between 35–45 mmHg and HCO_3 is 22–26 meq/L. In uncompensated respiratory acidosis pH is reduced, $PaCO_2$ is elevated and HCO_3 is normal.

ENT 1

1. G. Chronic otitis media

In this condition there is persistent drainage from the middle ear via a perforated tympanic membrane. The condition must be present for at least six weeks. Pain and fever are usually absent. On examination there is conductive hearing loss.

2. A. Acute mastoiditis

This is a severe bacterial infection which involves the mastoid part of the temporal bone and is a complication of acute otitis media. This requires prompt treatment.

3. K. Granulomatosis with polyangiitis

Previously known as Wegener's granulomatosis, this is a form of vasculitis which affects small and medium sized vessels. It commonly affects the ears, nose and throat as well as the respiratory system and the kidneys.

4. B. Acute otitis media

This is an infection which occurs in the middle ear behind the eardrum causing erythema and a bulging tympanic membrane. Treatment is initially to manage symptoms as most cases resolve spontaneously.

5. L. Nasal foreign body

These are common in children aged between two and five years and those with intellectual disabilities. Urgent ENT referral is required for button batteries and pair magnets as they can cause necrosis of tissue within the nose.

6. M. Otitis externa

Also known as swimmer's ear, this is an infection involving the external ear and is common in children who spend a great deal of time in water. In this condition there is pain with application of pressure to the tragus and pinna of the ear.

ENT 2

1. O. Rhinitis medicamentosa

The correct answer is Rhinitis medicamentosa. Also known as rebound congestion, this is a condition caused by overuse of nasal decongestants resulting in red and inflamed nasal mucosa.

2. N. Otitis media with effusion

This condition results from a collection of non-infective fluid within the middle ear. Patients may describe muffled hearing or a fullness within the ear. On examination this patient has a translucent tympanic membrane with reduced mobility and an air fluid level behind it. His exam findings are consistent with otitis media with effusion.

3. D. Allergic rhinitis

This patient has seasonal symptoms which are consistent with hay fever. This is an inflammatory condition in which the immune system of the body reacts disproportionately to allergens within the air.

4. F. Choanal atresia

Symptoms of bilateral choanal atresia usually present shortly after birth whereas unilateral choanal atresia typically presents later in life. Patients with unilateral choanal atresia commonly present with unilateral chronic rhinitis. This patient has imaging findings in keeping with choanal atresia.

5. E. Bullous myringitis

This is a painful condition in which bullae (blisters) form on the tympanic membrane. Bullous myringitis can be associated with hearing loss.

6. C. Acute rhinosinusitis

The acute form of rhinosinusitis lasts less than four weeks, chronic is defined as greater than 12 weeks.

Paediatric respiratory 1

1. N. Tracheo-Esophageal fistula

This condition can cause a newborn to passage fluid from the esophagus to the trachea which may result in respiratory infections.

2. O. Upper airway cough syndrome

Otherwise known as post-nasal drip, this condition occurs when there is excessive mucous production in the upper airways.

3. J. Peritonsillar abscess

This is a collection of pus between the affected tonsil and the superior pharyngeal constrictor muscle causing deviation of the uvula to the contralateral side. A peritonsillar abscess is a common complication of tonsillitis and is most commonly caused by group A streptococcal bacteria.

4. F. Influenza

Influenza has an incubation period of between one and four days and patients typically present with fever, sore throat, myalgia, rhinorrhoea, coughing and fatigue.

5. C. Bronchiolitis

Bronchiolitis is a viral respiratory infection most commonly caused by respiratory syncytial virus (RSV). The diagnosis is made on clinical grounds and is usually limited to the first 12 months of life. The presentation usually resolves within seven to ten days and does not require active treatment.

Paediatric respiratory 2

1. A. Acute epiglottitis.

This is a life-threatening presentation and the patient requires urgent escorted hospital transfer with airway management.

2. D. Croup

This is an acute upper respiratory illness characterised by a bark like cough. Parainfluenza viruses are the most common cause of croup. This patient has presented with a moderate form of croup and no investigations are required for diagnosis. For mild to moderate cases treatment involves minimal handling and oral steroids. Severe cases may require nebulised adrenaline and IV steroids.

3. L. Retropharyngeal abscess

This is a result of pus collection in the retropharyngeal region secondary to infection. Patients with this condition present with fever, odynophagia neck pain and or stiffness.

4. E. Infectious mononucleosis

Also known as glandular fever, this patient has presented with the most common symptoms. This condition is caused by a viral illness (Epstein–Barr virus).

5. M. Tonsillitis

This condition results from either bacterial or viral infection affecting the tonsils. Patients usually present in the acute phase with symptoms including swollen tonsils, tonsillar exudate, fever, fatigue, bad breath and dysphagia.

Paediatric respiratory 3

1. G. Inhaled foreign body

Children may have a history of coughing or choking while eating or playing. On examination some children may present with stridor (suggestive of partial upper airway obstruction), wheeze, decreased chest sounds or bronchial breath sounds.

2. K. Pulmonary sequestration

Also known as accessory lung, this is a condition in which a segment of lung exists without communication to the rest of the tracheobronchial tree.

3. I. Laryngomalacia

This is a congenital condition which involves softening of the larynx above the voice box.

4. B. Asthma

This is a condition in which the airways narrow, swell and produce excess mucus.

5. H. Laryngitis

This condition results from inflammation of the larynx, also known as the voice box. Patients typically present with hoarse voice, fever, dysphagia and pain.

Respiratory conditions 1

1. T. Sarcoidosis

This patient presents with sarcoidosis, a granulomatous inflammatory condition. The respiratory system is typically the most commonly affected part of the body, but there are other extrapulmonary manifestations of this condition such as erythema nodosum, lymphadenopathy and in this case lupus pernio.

2. R. Pulmonary aspergillosis

Failure to respond to broad spectrum antibiotics should raise suspicion about possibility of pulmonary aspergillosis. The halo sign represents a macro-nodule surrounded by a perimeter of ground glass opacity and is an early sign of invasive pulmonary aspergillosis.

3. B. Asthma

Patients with this condition suffer from respiratory symptoms as a result of airway narrowing secondary to inflammation and muscle tightening around the small airways. A trigger may be cold air at night.

4. Q. Pneumothorax

Also referred to as a collapsed lung, this condition results from air leakage into the pleural space between the lungs and the chest wall. If large enough, this causes a tension pneumothorax with mediastinal shift to the contralateral side.

5. H. Goodpasture syndrome

Also known as anti-glomerular basement disease, this is an autoimmune condition which affect the lungs and the kidneys. Diagnosis can be confirmed with renal biopsy showing IgG staining on the glomerular basement membrane.

6. G. Empyema

This is a collection of pus between the lung and the pleural space. The split pleura sign is typically seen on CT and helps distinguish between a lung abscess and empyema.

Respiratory conditions 2

1. U. Silicosis

Silicosis is an occupational lung disease caused by the inhalation of silica dust. Egg shell calcifications are well defined calcifications around the periphery of a lymph node (hilar or mediastinal) typically seen in silicosis. Sandblasting is a high-risk profession for development of silicosis.

2. L. Lobar pneumonia

This type of pneumonia affects one or more lobes of the lung. Auscultation normally reveals crackles, rales and bronchial breath sounds. There may also be dullness to percussion over the affected lobe or lobes.

3. F. Cystic fibrosis

This is a rare genetic disorder which causes damage to the respiratory and gastrointestinal systems. Patients may also have recurrent sinusitis and nasal polyps.

4. N. Lung adenocarcinoma

This is a type of non-small cell lung cancer and is the most common form of lung cancer in those who do not smoke.

5. M. Lung abscess

This is a pus-filled cavity in the chest that may arise as a complication of aspiration. It is typically round in shape on chest X-ray and contains an air-fluid level.

Respiratory conditions 3

1. S. Pulmonary embolism

This occurs when a blood clot obstructs an artery in the lung. Clots most commonly develop in the deep veins of the lower limbs and travel to the lungs via the right side of the heart. Malignancy and smoking are both risk factors for the development of a pulmonary embolism.

2. V. Tuberculosis

This is a respiratory infection which is caused by the bacteria *Mycobacterium tuberculosis*. While the lungs are most commonly affected, it can also affect other body systems. Cavitation on chest X-ray indicates advanced infection.

3. C. Bronchiectasis

Bronchiectasis is a condition marked by abnormal dilatation of the bronchial tree. Patients typically present with chronic cough and recurrent bronchial infections. Tram-Tracks on chest X-ray indicate cylindrical bronchiectasis.

4. I. Granulomatosis with polyangiitis

Previously known as Wegener's granulomatosis, this is a form of vasculitis which affects small and medium sized vessels. It is a multisystem disorder and c-ANCA is the most specific antibody test for this disease.

5. J. Haemothorax

This condition occurs when blood collects within the pleural cavity. Trauma is the cause in the case illustrated here.

Respiratory conditions 4

1. O. Mesothelioma

Mesothelioma is a form of lung cancer that results from prolonged exposure to and inhalation of asbestos. Fire fighters work in environments where there is a significant risk of asbestos exposure.

2. K. Idiopathic pulmonary fibrosis

This condition, also known as cryptogenic fibrosing alveolitis, results in inflammation and fibrosis of the alveoli and interstitium of the lungs. This patient has presented with worsening exertional shortness of breath, finger clubbing and restrictive pattern on spirometry.

3. E. Churg–Strauss syndrome

Also known as eosinophilic granulomatosis with polyangiitis. This is a condition in which there is abnormal clustering of white blood cells within the blood and tissues, granuloma formation and vasculitis. These patients also have asthma and chronic sinusitis.

4. D. Chronic obstructive airways disease

This patient has exam findings and imaging results consistent with a diagnosis of COPD. The spirometry reveals moderate obstructive changes.

5. A. Acute pulmonary oedema

This is a medical emergency which requires prompt treatment.

Pneumothorax

1. I. Tension pneumothorax

This patient has presented with a right sided tension pneumothorax secondary to blunt trauma. She is clinically unstable with tachypnoea, tachycardia, hypotension and hypoxaemia. This is a medical emergency and she requires immediate needle decompression followed by an intercostal catheter.

2. B. Chylothorax

This results from the accumulation of chyle in the pleural space, in this particular post-surgical case. Malignancies are also the most common cause of unilateral pleural effusion.

3. H. Secondary spontaneous pneumothorax

This patient has presented with a secondary spontaneous pneumothorax. There is no precipitating event and COPD can be a very common cause for secondary spontaneous pneumothorax.

4. A. Catamenial pneumothorax

This is a form of spontaneous pneumothorax that occurs within 72 hours of menstruation. It most commonly occurs on the right side and are usually small or moderately sized. Some catamenial pneumothoraces can occur due to thoracic endometriosis.

5. G. Primary spontaneous pneumothorax

This patient has presented with a primary spontaneous pneumothorax. There is no precipitating event and he has no history of underlying lung disease. Patients may delay seeking medical review for several days after onset of symptoms.

Occupational respiratory conditions 1

1. I. Psittacosis

This condition is also known as ornithosis or bird fancier's lung. It is caused by the bacterium *Chlamydia psittaci* which is carried by birds. Humans can be at risk of contracting this condition by contact with bird droppings or feathers.

2. H. Occupational asthma

Isocyanate paints create a fine airborne mist which can lead to the development of occupational asthma.

3. A. Asbestosis

Fire fighters have a very high risk of asbestos exposure. This patient's history, occupation and chest X-ray findings are suggestive of asbestosis.

4. E. Coal workers pneumoconiosis

Also known as black lung disease, this condition is caused by the inhalation of coal dust which leads to scarring of the lungs and associated respiratory symptoms.

5. B. Bronchiolitis obliterans

Also known as popcorn workers lung, this is a syndrome affecting the small airways. Exposure to diacetyl, which is used in the production of microwave popcorn, has been associated with this condition.

Occupational respiratory conditions 2

1. F. Hypersensitivity pneumonitis

Also known as farmer's lung, this condition results from inhalation of biologic dusts which cause an inflammatory response within the lungs.

2. D. Byssinosis

This condition is a respiratory illness that results from cotton dust exposure.

3. K. Silicosis

Silicosis is an occupational lung disease caused by the inhalation of silica dust. Egg shell calcifications are well defined calcifications around the periphery of a lymph node (hilar or mediastinal) typically seen in silicosis. Sandblasting is a high-risk profession for development of silicosis.

4. G. Legionnaires' disease
This is a severe form of pneumonia most commonly caused by *Legionella pneumophila*. The bacteria can contaminate cooling towers of large air conditioners and pose an occupational risk for people who service them.

5. C. Brucellosis
Most cases of brucellosis associated with unpasteurised milk are caused by *Brucella abortus* and *Brucella melitensis*. It is endemic in some Mediterranean countries, the Middle East, Sub-Saharan Africa, Central Asia and Central and Southern Latin America.

Lung cancer

1. D. Lung adenocarcinoma
The lesion is not visualised on bronchoscopy and it is therefore located in the lung periphery. Lung adenocarcinoma is the most common type of lung cancer in non-smokers.

2. G. Pancoast tumor
This type of cancer forms in the apex of the lung, it can result in shoulder pain and upper limb neuropathy as a result of invasion of the brachial plexus.

3. A. Bronchial carcinoid
Bronchial carcinoids are highly vascular and may appear as cherry red nodules on bronchoscopy.

4. H. Small cell lung carcinoma
This is an aggressive form of lung cancer which commonly affects smokers. The presence of hyponatraemia occurs because of ectopic antidiuretic hormone production by tumour cells.

5. F. Mesothelioma
Mesothelioma is a form of lung cancer that results from prolonged exposure to and inhalation of asbestos. Pipe laggers work in environments where there is a significant risk of asbestos exposure.

Chest imaging findings 1

1. F. Left atrial enlargement
Also known as the double right heart border, this sign is seen when there is left atrial enlargement. The right side of the left atrium extends behind the right cardiac shadow creating its own silhouette.

2. J. Pleural effusion
This sign usually indicates a small pleural effusion.

3. M. Pneumothorax
This is caused by the air in the pleural cavity which outlines the anterior costophrenic angle and the aerated lung which outlines the diaphragmatic dome.

4. K. Pleural empyema
Split pleura sign on chest CT can help distinguish an empyema from an abscess.

5. P. Sarcoidosis
This sign describes a cluster of tiny round nodules measuring 1–2 mm each which are distributed uniformly in all or part of a lymph node.

6. B. Asbestosis
These are calcified pleural plaques which give the appearance of holly leaves. Pleural plaques are a common finding amongst those who have been exposed to asbestos.

7. G. Lobar consolidation
This sign is classically associated with right upper lobe consolidation.

Chest imaging findings 2

1. I. Pericardial effusion
This sign is as a result of gradual stretching of the pericardium, as a result of an effusion, causing it to appear saggy like an old-fashioned water bottle.

2. A. Acute pulmonary edema
The most common reason for this sign is the accumulation of oedema fluid in the lungs.

3. O. Round atelectasis
This is a curvilinear opacity which extends towards the ipsilateral hilum from a subpleural mass. It results from distortion of the bronchi and vessels which lead to an area of round atelectasis, the mass.

4. Q. Tetralogy of Fallot
This sign is as a result of an upturned apex of the heart secondary to right ventricular hypertrophy and a concave pulmonary artery segment.

5. S. Transposition of the great arteries
This sign occurs as a result of the cardio mediastinal silhouette seen with transposition of the great arteries.

6. C. Bronchiectasis
The ring represents the wall of a dilated bronchus and a smaller opacity representing its pulmonary artery.

Chest imaging findings 3

1. E. Coarctation of the aorta
This sign if formed by the aortic knuckle, the stenotic portion of the aorta and the dilated post-stenotic segment of the descending aorta.

2. R. Total anomalous pulmonary venous return
This sign refers to the configuration of the heart and the superior mediastinal border. It is also called the figure of eight sign.

3. D. Chronic obstructive airways disease
This finding is pathognomonic for COPD. It refers to coronal narrowing of the trachea intrathoracically and associated sagittal widening.

4. L. Pneumomediastinum
This occurs when there is lucency seen above the diaphragm. This is highly suggestive of free gas in the mediastinum.

5. **N. Pulmonary embolism**

This sign describes a dilated and prominent central pulmonary artery which can be caused by pulmonary hypertension chronically or a large pulmonary embolism which acutely enlarges the luminal diameter of the proximal artery.

6. **H. Lung abscess**

This is the classical radiographic finding of a lung abscess.

Respiratory microbiology 1

1. **E. Legionella pneumophila**

This patient has presented with Legionnaires' disease, a severe form of pneumonia most commonly caused by *Legionella pneumophila*. These bacteria can contaminate cooling towers of large air conditioners and pose an occupational risk for people who service them.

2. **H. Pneumocystis jirovecii**

Pneumocystis jirovecii pneumonia (PJP) is an infection which frequently affects immunocompromised individuals, particularly people with HIV or AIDS.

3. **L. Streptococcus pyogenes**

This patient has presented with scarlet fever. Patients typically present with a fever, sore throat, lymphadenopathy, myalgia and malaise. The rash usually commences within 48 hours of commencement of fever and can feel like rough sand paper.

4. **J. Staphylococcus aureus**

Multiple lung abscesses on chest X-ray indicate that *Staphylococcus aureus* is the most likely organism behind this presentation.

5. **D. Haemophilus influenzae**

This patient has presented with bronchiectasis, a condition marked by abnormal dilatation of the bronchial tree. Patients typically present with chronic cough and recurrent bronchial infections. *Haemophilus influenza* is one of the most common organisms found to colonise damaged bronchi.

Respiratory microbiology 2

1. **K. Streptococcus pneumoniae**

This patient has presented with a case of community acquired pneumonia (CAP). This type of pneumonia affects one or more lobes of the lung. Auscultation normally reveals crackles, rales and bronchial breath sounds. There may also be dullness to percussion over the affected lobe or lobes. The most common organism to cause this infection is *Streptococcus pneumoniae*.

2. **F. Mycoplasma pneumoniae**

This patient likely has *Mycoplasma pneumoniae* and her symptoms are less severe than a typical lower respiratory tract infection. These patients also have concurrent upper respiratory tract symptoms and occasionally extrapulmonary manifestations such as haemolysis.

3. I. Pseudomonas aeruginosa

This is a common cause of lung infections if patients with cystic fibrosis.

4. C. Chlamydia psittaci

This patient has presented with psittacosis also known as ornithosis or bird fancier's lung. It is caused by the bacterium *Chlamydia psittaci* which is carried by birds. Humans can be at risk of contracting this condition by contact with bird droppings or feathers.

5. B. Bordetella pertussis

This patient is unvaccinated and has paroxysmal coughs post coughing which suggests infection with *Bordetella pertussis*.

6. G. Mycoplasma tuberculosis

The correct answer is *Mycoplasma tuberculosis*.

Index

A

abdomen, cramping/pain, 1, 2, 3, 10, 16
ABO blood group, incompatibility of, 20, 30
absence seizure, 86, 102
acanthosis nigricans, 47, 54
accessory lung, 237
accessory spinal nerve, 83, 101
achalasia, 6, 24, 26
Achilles tendon rupture, 159, 178
acrolentiginous melanoma, 38, 50
acromegaly, 196, 206
actinic keratoses, 44, 53
acute angle closure glaucoma, 99, 107
acute compartment syndrome, 159, 178
acute dystonia, 95, 106
acute epiglottitis, 216, 236
acute generalised exanthematous pustulosis, 35, 49
acute interstitial nephritis, 153, 157
acute mastoiditis, 213, 235
acute myocardial infarction, 176, 186
acute otitis media, 92, 104, 213, 235
acute paronychia, 37, 50
acute pericarditis, 193, 205
acute post-streptococcal glomerulonephritis, 152, 156
acute pulmonary edema, 223–224, 230, 239, 242
acute rhinosinusitis, 88, 103, 215, 236
acute stress disorder, 60, 76
acute tubular necrosis, 152, 156
addictive disorders, *see* substance related and addictive disorders
Addisonian crisis, 190, 204
adenomyosis, 115–116, 137
adhesive capsulitis, 176, 186
adjustment disorder, 61, 77
adjustment sleep disorder, 59, 76
age related macular degeneration (ARMD), 107
agoraphobia, 61, 77
Alcock canal syndrome, 151, 156
alcoholic hepatitis, 14, 28
alcohol intoxication, 71, 81
alcohol withdrawal, 71, 81
allergic contact dermatitis, 40, 51, 121, 139
allergic rhinitis, 214, 235
alopecia areata, 36, 49
amaurosis fugax, 99, 107

amenorrhoea, 109–110, 135
amniotic fluid embolism, 125, 141
amphetamine intoxication, 72, 81
amyloidosis, 210
anabolic steroids, 138
anal fissure, 18, 29
Angelman syndrome, 132, 144
angina pectoris, 187, 203
angiokeratoma of Fordyce, 150, 156
ankle and shin disorders, 159–160, 178–179
ankylosing spondylitis, 107, 162, 179
anorexia nervosa, 74, 82, 110, 135
answers
    amenorrhoea, 135
    ankle and shin, 178–179
    anxiety, 76–77
    arrhythmias, 205–206
    arterial blood gas interpretation, 234
    back pain, 179
    behavioural conditions, 77–78
    bowel conditions, 22–23
    breast pathology, 136–137
    cardiac structure, 209–210
    cardiac vessels, 203
    CHA2DS2-VASc Scoring, 208
    chest imaging findings, 241–243
    chest pain, 203
    childhood infections, 48
    collapse, 204
    complications of pregnancy, 139
    cranial nerve pathology, 101
    dermatitis, 51
    dizziness, 101–102
    dysmenorrhoea, 142
    eating disorders, 81–82
    elbow and forearm, 180–181
    ENT, 234–236
    epilepsy, 102–103
    esophageal disorders, 23–24
    facial pain, 103
    female infertility, 140–141
    foot pain, 181–182
    gastric disorders, 24–25
    gastrointestinal conditions (paediatric), 25–26
    gastrointestinal imaging, 26–27
    genetic disorders, 143–144
    hair, 49

hand and wrist, 182–184
headache, 103–104
hearing loss, 104–105
heart failure grading, 209
hepatobiliary disease, 27–28
hip pain, 184–185
hypertension, 206
hypertension grading, 208–209
inflammatory disorders, 52
knee pain, 185–186
lumps and hernias, 28–29
lung cancer, 241
male infertility, 138
memory, 78–79
menstrual irregularities, 137–138
mood disorders, 75
movement disorders, 105–106
murmurs, 207–208
nails, 50
nail signs of systemic illness, 50–51
neck and shoulder pain, 186
neuromuscular disorders, 106
obstetric complications, 141–142
occupational respiratory conditions, 240–241
paediatric jaundice, 30–31
paediatric respiratory, 236–237
paraphilic conditions, 79–80
pelvic-abdominal pain, 144–145
penis disorders, 154
perianal conditions, 29–30
personality disorders, 80
pigmentation disorders, 53–54
pneumothorax, 239–240
respiratory conditions, 237–239
respiratory microbiology, 243–244
sexually transmitted infection, 142–143
skin lesions, 52–53
skin reactions, 48–49
sleep disturbances, 75–76
substance related and addictive disorders, 80–81
testicular and scrotal disorders, 154–156
urology, 156–157
vision loss, 107
vulvovaginal pathology, 139, 140
anterior cruciate ligament tear, 174, 185
Anterior drawer test, 178
anterior talo-fibular ligament injury (ATFL), 160,
    178–179
anti-gliadin antibodies, 7
anti-glomerular basement disease, 238
antisocial personality disorder, 62, 69, 77, 80
anxiety, 60–61, 76–77
aorta, coarctation of, 195, 206, 231, 242
aortic regurgitation, 196, 207
apparent leukonychia, 39, 50
appendicitis, 9, 25, 133, 144

apple core sign, 11, 26
arrhythmias, 81, 192–194, 205
arterial blood gas interpretation, 211–212, 234
arteries, 189, 203
arteritis
    giant cell, 107
    temporal, 88–89, 103
arthritis
    psoriatic, 169, 183
    rheumatoid, 171, 183
    septic, 175, 186
arthropathy, 183
asbestosis, 226, 229, 240, 242
ascending cholangitis, 16, 28
Asherman's syndrome, 124, 141
asteatotic dermatitis, 40, 51
asthma, 6, 218, 219, 237
    occupational, 226, 240
atopic dermatitis, 41, 51
atrial fibrillation, 192, 205
atrial myxoma, 196, 207
atrial septal defect, 200, 209
atrophic vaginitis, 121–122, 140
attention deficit hyperactivity disorder (ADHD),
    62, 77
auscultation, 238
autism spectrum disorder, 63, 78
avascular necrosis of navicular bone, 182
avoidant personality disorder, 68, 80
avoidant restrictive food intake disorder, 73, 81

B

back pain, 161–163, 179
bacterial vaginosis, 129, 142
Baker's cyst, ruptured, 174, 185
balanitis xerotica obliterans, 147, 154
barium swallow, 6, 7, 12, 24
Barlow syndrome, 210
barotrauma, 92, 104
Barrett's esophagus, 5, 23
Bartholin's cyst, 121, 139
Basal cell carcinoma, 44, 53
Beau's lines, 39, 51
behavioural disorders, 62–63, 77–78
Bell's palsy, 96, 106
benign paroxysmal positional vertigo (BPPV),
    85, 102
biceps, long head of rupture, 176, 186
biceps tendinitis, 177, 186
biliary atresia, 21, 31
binge eating disorder, 73, 82
biopsy, 6, 7, 42
bipolar disorder, 57, 75
bird fancier's lung, 240
bird's beak sign, 12, 26

black lung disease, 240
black pearls sign, cluster of, 229, 242
bleeding
    dysfunctional uterine, 115, 138
    rectal, 2
blighted ovum, 119, 139
bloating, 4
body dysmorphic disorder, 61, 77
borderline personality disorder, 62, 77
Bordetella pertussis, 244
Bouchard's nodes, 183
bowel disease, 1–4, 22–23
bowel obstruction, 1–2, 22
bowel perforation, 3, 23
Bowen's disease, 53
boxer's muscle, 186
breast abscess, 113, 136
breast cyst, 112, 136
breast disorders, 112–113, 136–137
breast lymphoma, 112, 136
breast milk jaundice, 21, 31
bronchial carcinoids, 228, 241
bronchiectasis, 222, 230, 232, 238, 242, 243
bronchiolitis, 216, 236
bronchiolitis obliterans, 226, 240
bronchoscopy, 228
Brown–Sequard syndrome, 161, 179
Brucella abortus, 241
Brucella melitensis, 241
brucellosis, 227, 241
bulging fissure sign, 229, 242
bulimia nervosa, 74, 82
bullous myringitis, 215, 235
byssinosis, 227, 240

C

caffeine intoxication, 72, 81
calcaneal apophysitis, 181
calcaneal petechiae, 181
calcium pyrophosphate crystals, 182
cancer
    endometrial, 114, 137
    esophageal, 5, 23
    gastric, 7, 24
    lung, *see* lung cancer
    pancreatic, 13, 27
candidal intertrigo, 150, 155
candida onychia, 38, 50
candidiasis, 130, 143
cannabis intoxication, 71, 81
capitellum, 180
carcinoid syndrome, 3, 22
cardiac tamponade, 191, 192, 205
cardiac vessels, 189, 203
cardiovascular diseases, 198–200, 209

carpal tunnel syndrome, 171, 184
carpenter's knee, 185
Carvallo's sign, 207
catamenial pneumothorax, 225, 240
caterpillar sign, 11, 26
cauda equina syndrome, 162–163, 179
central retinal artery occlusion (CRAO), 99, 107
central retinal vein occlusion (CRVO), 98, 107
cephalohematoma, 20, 30
cerumen impaction, 93, 105
cervical ectropion, 114, 137
cervical stenosis, 128, 142
CHA_2DS_2-VASc scoring, 198, 208
charcot arthropathy, 159, 178
Charcot–Marie–Tooth disease, 97, 107
Charcot's triad, 28
chest pain, 6, 187–188, 203
chicken pox, 32, 48
chilblains, 169, 183
children
    jaundice in, *see* paediatric jaundice
    respiratory diseases in, *see* pediatric respiratory
        conditions
    skin infections in, *see* skin infections, in children
Chlamydia psittaci, 240, 244
chlamydia trachomatis, 128–129, 142
chloasma, 54
choanal atresia, 214, 235
cholecystitis, 13, 27
choledocholithiasis, 13, 27
cholesteatoma, 92, 105
chondrodermatitis nodularis helicis, 45, 53
chorioamnionitis, 119, 139
chronic obstructive airways disease (COPD), 223,
        231, 239, 242
chronic otitis media, 213, 234–235
chronic paronychia, 38, 50
chronic prostatitis, 153, 157
Churg–Strauss syndrome, 223, 239
chylothorax, 224, 239
Clostridium difficile, 23
cluster headache, 90, 104
coal workers pneumoconiosis, 226, 240
coarctation of aorta, 231, 242
cocaine intoxication, 70, 80
coeliac disease, 7, 24
coffee bean sign, 12, 26
collapse, 190–191, 204
collapsed lung, 237
colonoscopy, 1, 4, 23
colorectal carcinoma, 11, 26
comet tail sign, 230, 242
community acquired pneumonia (CAP), 233, 243
complete miscarriage, 120, 139
complex partial seizure, 87, 102
conduct disorder, 63, 78

condyloma, 18, 29
condyloma acuminata, 121, 140
congenital adrenal hyperplasia (CAH), 109–110, 135
Conn's syndrome, 206
constipation, 4
continuous diaphragm sign, 231, 242
corkscrew appearance, 12, 27
cornual pregnancy, 120, 139
Corrigan's pulse, 207
corticosteroids, 24
Corynebacterium minutissimum, 53
cottage loaf sign, 12, 26
Coxsackie virus, 48
cramping, abdominal, 2, 3
cranial nerve pathology, 83–84, 101
crepitus, 180
CREST (calcinosis cutis, Raynaud phenomenon,
    esophageal dysmotility, sclerodactyly and
    telangiectasia), 182
Crohn's disease, 1, 22, 27
croup, 216–217, 236
cryptorchidism, 116–117, 138
cubital tunnel syndrome, 164, 180
Cushing syndrome, 110, 122–123, 135, 140
cutaneous fibrous histiocytoma, 52
cystic fibrosis, 9, 25, 220–221, 238
cystitis, 152, 156

D

dactylitis (sausage finger), 183
deep vein thrombosis (DVT), 160, 178
Del Castillo syndrome, 116–117, 138
delusional disorder, 57, 75
dementia
    frontotemporal, 64, 78
    lewy body, 66, 79
    vascular, 64, 78
de Musset's sign, 207
dependent personality disorder, 69, 80
De Quervain's tenosynovitis, 163, 180
dermatillomania, 61, 77
dermatitis, 40–41, 51, 121, 139
dermatofibroma, 44, 53
dermatological diseases, *see* skin diseases
diabetic neuropathy, 190, 204
diaphragmatic rupture, 27
diarrhoea, 1, 2, 3, 4
diffuse esophageal spasm, 6, 24, 27
digital rectal examination, 10
dilated cardiomyopathy, 201, 209
direct inguinal hernia, 17, 29
discoid eczema, 51
disruptive mood dysregulation disorder, 55, 75
dissecting thoracic aortic aneurysm, 161, 179,
    188, 203
distal interphalangeal (DIP) joints, 170, 183

divarication of recti, 16, 28
diverticulitis, 4, 23
dizziness, 84–85, 101–102
double bubble sign, 11, 26
double density sign, 229, 241
double diaphragm sign, 229, 241
Down syndrome, 10, 26, 130, 143
DRESS syndrome, 34, 48
drug induced infertility, 118, 138
Duchenne muscular dystrophy, 97, 106
ductal carcinoma in situ (DCIS), 112, 136
ductal ectasia, 112, 136
dumping syndrome, 7, 24
duodenal atresia, 10, 26
duodenal ulcers, 8, 25
duodenum, biopsy of, 7
Dupuytren's disease, 169, 182
dysfunctional uterine bleeding, 115, 138
dyshidrotic eczematous dermatitis, 41, 51
dysmenorrhoea, 127–128, 142
dysphagia, 6, 182
dystrophin, 106

E

eating disorders, 73–74, 81–82
Ebstein's anomaly, 202, 210
eclampsia, 125, 141
ectopic pregnancy, 126, 128, 142
eczema, 6, 51
    nummular, 41, 51
elbow and forearm disorders, 163–165, 180–181
electrocution, 186
electromyography, 96
empyema, 219, 238
endometrial cancer, 114, 137
endometriosis, 114–115, 124, 127, 133, 137, 141,
    142, 144
endoscopy, 7, 23, 24, *see also* gastroscopy
ENT disorders, 212–215, 234–236
eosinophilic esophagitis, 6, 24
eosinophilic granulomatosis with polyangiitis, 239
epididymis, 154
epigastric hernias, 17, 29
epiglottitis, acute, 216, 236
epilepsy, 85–87, 102
epileptic seizure, 191, 204
epispadias, 146–147, 154
Epstein–Barr virus, 236
erythema infectiosum, 32, 48
erythema multiforme, 43, 52
erythema nodosum, 43, 52
erythrasma, 46, 53
esophageal cancer, 5, 23
esophageal candidiasis, 6, 24
esophageal varices, 5, 24
esophagus disorders, 5–6, 23–24, 26

essential tremor, 94, 105
eustachian tube dysfunction, 93, 105
exhibitionistic disorder, 68, 80
exostosis, 93, 105

F

facial nerve, 83, 101
facial pain, 88–89, 103
factor X deficiency, 115, 137
farmer's lung, 240
fat necrosis, 112, 136
febrile seizure, 85–86, 102
female infertility, 122–124, 140–141
female sexual health disorders, 108–116
femoral hernia, 17, 29
fetishistic disorder, 66, 79
fever, 3, 9, 14
    rheumatic, 33, 48
fibroadenoma, 111, 136
fibroids, 127, 142
figure 3 sign, 231, 242
Finkelstein test, 163, 180
first-degree heart block, 192, 205
fixed drug eruption, 35, 49
flamingo pink blush, 104
flatulence, 4
Fleischner sign, 231, 243
folliculitis, 122, 140
foot pain, 165–168, 181–182
forearm disorders, *see* elbow and forearm disorders
foreign body
    inhaled, 218, 237
    nasal, 213, 235
Fournier's gangrene, 150–151, 156
fracture
    penile, 146, 154
    spinal compression, 162, 179
    stress, 168, 182
fragile X syndrome, 131, 143
Freiberg disease, 165, 181
frontotemporal dementia, 64, 78
frotteuristic disorder, 67, 79

G

galactocele, 113, 137
galactosaemia, 20, 30
galeazzi test, 184
gastric cancer, 7, 24
gastric disorders, 7–8, 24–25
gastric ulcer, 8, 25
gastrocnemius tear, 160, 178
gastroenteritis, 8, 9, 25
gastroesophageal reflux disease, 6, 24
gastrointestinal imaging, 11–12, 26–27
gastroscopy, 5, 6, *see also* endoscopy

generalised anxiety disorder, 60, 77
genetic disorders, 130–132, 143–144
genital herpes, 129, 143
genital psoriasis, 120, 139
giant cell arteritis, 107
Gilbert's syndrome, 16, 28
glandular fever, 236
glossopharyngeal nerve, 84, 101
glucose hydrogen breath test, 4, 23
golfer's elbow, 181
gonorrhoea, 129, 143
goodpasture syndrome, 219, 238
gout, 166, 181
G6PD deficiency, 21, 31
granuloma annulare, 42, 52
granulomatosis with polyangiitis, 213, 222, 235, 239
    eosinophilic, 239
greater occipital neuralgia, 89, 103
growing pain, 166, 181
gumma of the testis, 148, 155

H

haematemesis, 5
haemochromatosis, 16, 28, 171, 183
Haemophilus influenzae, 243
haemorrhage
    postpartum, 126, 142
    subarachnoid, 91, 104
haemorrhoids, internal, 18, 29
haemothorax, 222, 239
hair diseases, 36, 49
hallux valgus, 168, 182
Haloperidol, 94, 95, 105, 106
halo sign, 237
hammer toe, 168, 182
hand, foot and mouth disease, 32, 48
hand and wrist disorders, 169–171, 182–183
Hashimoto's thyroiditis, 123–124, 140
headaches, 89–90, 103–104
hearing loss, 92–93, 104–105
heart block
    first-degree, 192, 205
    second-degree-Mobitz type 2, 192–193, 205
    third-degree, 194, 205
heart diseases, *see* cardiovascular diseases
heart failure grading, 199–200, 209
Heberden's nodes, 183
heel fat pad syndrome, 165, 181
Helicobacter pylori, 25
Henoch–Schönlein purpura, 148, 154
Hepatitis A, 14, 27–28
Hepatitis B
    acute, 13–14, 27
    chronic, 13, 27
    resolved, 14–15, 28
hepatobiliary diseases, 13–16, 27–28

hernias, 7, 16–17, 28–29, 172, 184
herpes simplex virus, 143
Hiatus hernia, 7, 24
high attenuating crescent sign, 11, 26
hip pain, 172–173, 184
Hirschsprung's disease, 10, 26
hirsutism, 36, 49
histrionic personality disorder, 68, 80
holly leaf sign, 229
Hortaea werneckii, 53
human papillomavirus, 129, 143
Huntington's disease, 65–66, 79, 94, 105
hydatidiform mole, 119, 139
hydrocele, 148, 155
hyperinsulinemia, 206
hyperprolactinaemia, 118, 124, 138, 141
hypersensitivity pneumonitis, 227, 240
hypertension, 8, 30, 194–196, 206, 208–209
hypertrichosis, 36, 49
hypertrophic cardiomyopathy (HOCM), 191, 193,
    204, 205
hypnic myoclonus, 87, 102
hypoglycaemia, 24
hypoglycaemic episode, 190, 204
hypogonadotrophic hypogonadism, 122, 140
hypoplastic left heart syndrome, 202, 210
hypospadias, 146, 154
hypothyroidism, 21, 30, 109, 115, 135, 138, 196, 206

I

ibuprofen, 8, 115, 160
ice pick headache, 89, 103
idiopathic intracranial hypertension, 90, 104
idiopathic pulmonary fibrosis, 223, 239
iliotibial band syndrome, 174, 185
impending abdominal aortic aneurysm rupture, 26
inclusion body myositis, 96, 106
indirect inguinal hernia, 17, 29
inevitable miscarriage, 119, 139
infectious mononucleosis, 217, 236
infertility
    female, *see* female infertility
    male, *see* male infertility
inflammatory skin diseases, 42–43, 51–52
influenza, 216, 236
inguinal hernia, 172, 184
    direct, 17, 29
    indirect, 17, 29
inhaled foreign body, 218, 237
internal haemorrhoid, 18, 29
intersection syndrome, 163, 180
intussusception, 9, 25, 27
invasive squamous cell carcinoma, 45, 53
iritis, 99, 107
irritable bowel syndrome, 2, 22
irritant contact dermatitis, 41, 51

ischaemic colitis, 3, 22
isocyanate paints, 240
isolated systolic hypertension, 199, 208

J

Jarisch-Herxheimer reaction, 35, 49
jaundice, paediatric, *see* paediatric jaundice
javelin throwers elbow, 180
jock itch, 155
jumper's knee, 185
juvenile myoclonic epilepsy (JME), 86, 102

K

Kallmann syndrome, 109–110, 117, 135, 138
Kawasaki syndrome, 33, 48
keratitis, 98, 107
keratoacanthoma, 44, 52
Kernig's sign, 91, 104
Kleine–Levin syndrome, 74, 82
kleptomania, 63, 78
Klinefelter syndrome (XXY), 117, 131, 138, 144
knee pain, 174–175, 185–186
Koenen tumors, 50
Kohler disease, 168, 182
koilonychia, 39, 50

L

labyrinthitis, 84, 101
lactating adenoma, 111, 136
large bowel obstruction, 1, 22
laryngitis, 218, 237
laryngomalacia, 218, 237
lateral epicondylitis, 164, 180
lead pipe sign, 12, 27
left anterior descending artery, 189, 204
left atrial enlargement, 229, 241
left circumflex artery, 189, 203
Legionella pneumophila, 241, 243
Legionnaires' disease, 227, 231, 241, 243
leiomyomas, 137
lewy body dementia, 66, 79
lichen planus, 42, 52
lichen sclerosus, 120, 139
lichen simplex chronicus, 40, 51
lobar consolidation, 229, 242
lobar pneumonia, 220, 238
long thoracic nerve palsy, 176, 186
low CSF headache, 90, 103
lumps, and hernias, 16–17, 28–29
lung abscess, 221, 231, 238, 243
lung adenocarcinoma, 221, 228, 238, 241
lung cancer
    bronchial carcinoids, 228, 241
    lung adenocarcinoma, 221, 228, 238, 241

mesothelioma, 228, 241
pancoast tumor, 228, 241
small cell, 228, 241

M

macular degeneration, 99, 107
major depressive disorder, 56–57, 75
male infertility, 116–118, 138
malingering, 63, 78
mallet toe, 165, 181
Mallory-Weiss tears, 5, 23
mammography, 136
Marfan syndrome, 130, 143
mask of pregnancy, 54
mastitis, 111, 136
measles, 33, 48
Meckel's diverticulum, 2, 22
meconium ileus, 9, 25
medial epicondylitis, 165, 181
median nerve palsy, 169, 183
medication overuse headache, 90–91, 104
melasma, 47, 54
memory disorders, 64–66, 78–79
meningitis, 91, 104
meniscal tear, 175, 185
menopause, 110, 135
menstrual irregularities, 114–116, 137–138
meralgia paraesthetica, 173, 184
mesenteric adenitis, 10, 26
mesothelioma, 223, 228, 239, 241
metabolic acidosis – uncompensated, 211, 234
metabolic alkalosis – partially compensated,
    211, 234
migraine, vestibular, 84, 101
migraine with aura, 91, 104
miscarriage, 119–120, 139
mitral regurgitation, 197, 207
mitral stenosis, 197, 207
mitral valve prolapse, 201, 210
mittelschmerz, 132, 144
molluscum contagiosum, 19, 30, 32–33, 48, 122, 140
molluscum sebaceum, 52
Mondor disease, 111, 136
monkey muscle tear, 178
mood disorders, 55–57, 75
morphea, 43, 52
Morton's neuroma, 168, 182
motor neurone disease, 97, 106
movement disorders, 94–95, 105–106
Mulder's click test, 168, 182
multiple myeloma, 161, 179
multiple sclerosis (MS), 96, 106
mumps, 34, 48
murmurs, 196–198, 207
Murphy's sign, 13, 27
myasthenia gravis, 97, 106

Mycobacterium tuberculosis, 238
Mycoplasma pneumoniae, 243
Mycoplasma tuberculosis, 244
myocardial infarction, 189, 203
myoclonic seizures, 102
myxoid cyst, 37, 50

N

nails, and signs of systemic illness, 39, 50–51
nails diseases 37–38, 49–50
narcissistic personality disorder, 70, 80
narcolepsy, 58, 76
nasal foreign body, 213, 235
nausea, 14
neck and shoulder pain, 176–177, 186
neck of femur fracture, 172, 184
necrotising enterocolitis, 10, 26
Neisseria gonorrhoeae, 143
neonatal seizures, 87, 103
nephroblastoma, 25, 157
nerves, 83–84, 101
neuroleptic malignant syndrome, 94, 105
neuromuscular disorders, 96–97, 106–107
neurosyphilis, 65, 78–79
night eating syndrome, 73, 82
Nikolsky sign, 34
nipple thrush, 112, 136
nipple vasospasm, 113, 137
nitrazine paper test, 125, 141
nonopioid analgesia, 104
Noonan syndrome, 131, 143
normal pressure hydrocephalus, 64, 78
NYHA Class II, heart failure grading, 200, 209
NYHA Class III, heart failure grading, 200, 209
NYHA Class IV, heart failure grading,
    199–200, 209

O

obsessive compulsive disorder, 61, 77
obstetric complications, 125–127, 141–142
obstructive sleep apnoea, 59, 76, 194, 206
occupational asthma, 226, 240
occupational respiratory conditions, 226–227,
    240–241
oesophageal spasm, 188, 203
Ogilvie syndrome, 3, 22
olecranon bursitis, 164, 180
olfactory nerve, 83–84, 101
onychogryphosis, 38, 50
onycholysis, 38, 50
opioids, 104
opioid withdrawal, 72, 81
oppositional defiant disorder, 62, 77
optimal blood pressure, 199, 208
ornithosis, 240

orthorexia nervosa, 74, 82
Osgood–Schlatter disease, 175, 185
osteitis pubis, 172, 184
osteoarthritis, 8, 170, 183
osteoid osteoma, 160, 178
otic barotrauma, 104
otitis externa, 93, 105, 213, 235
otitis media, 213–214, 234–235
otosclerosis, 92, 104
ototoxicity, 92, 104
ovarian hyperstimulation syndrome, 133, 144
ovarian torsion, 133–134, 144
ovulation pain, 144

P

paediatric jaundice, 20–21, 30–31
paedophilic disorder – exclusive type, 67, 79
Paget's disease, 113, 136
panchyonychia congenita, 37, 50
pancoast tumor, 228, 241
pancreatic cancer, 13, 27
pancreatitis, 15, 28
panic attack, 61, 77, 84, 101, 191, 204
Panner's disease, 163, 180
papilloma, 113–114, 137
paracetamol, 8, 91, 178
parainfluenza viruses, 236
paranoid personality disorder, 68, 80
paraphilic disorders, 66–68, 79–80
paraphimosis, 146, 154
paraumbilical hernia, 17, 29
Parkinsonism, 94, 105
Parkinson's disease, 65, 79, 95, 96, 106
paronychia
    acute, 37, 50
    chronic, 38, 50
patellar tendinopathy, 174, 185
patellofemoral pain syndrome, 175, 185
pediatric gastrointestinal disorders, 9–10, 25–26
pediatric respiratory conditions, 216–218, 236–237
pelvic-abdominal pain, 132–134, 144–145
pelvic inflammatory disease, 128, 134, 142, 145
penile fracture, 146, 154
penile Mondor's disease, 147, 154
penis disorders, 146–147, 154
perforated peptic ulcer, 8, 25
perforation, of bowel, 3, 23
perianal abscess, 19, 30
perianal conditions/diseases, 18–19, 29–30
perianal haematoma, 19, 30
pericardial effusion, 230, 242
pericarditis, 188, 197–198, 203, 207
periodic limb movement disorder, 58, 76
peripartum cardiomyopathy, 201, 209
peritonsillar abscess, 215–216, 236

periungual fibroma, 39, 51
perniosis, 183
personality disorders, 62, 68–70, 77, 80
Perthes disease, 173, 185
phencyclidine (PCP) intoxication, 71, 81
phimosis, 146, 154
phyllodes tumor, 111, 136
physiological jaundice, 20, 30
pica, 73, 81
pigmentation disorders, 46–47, 53–54
pilar cyst, 44, 52
pilonidal sinus, 18, 29
pitcher's elbow, 180
pityriasis alba, 47, 54
pityriasis rosea, 43, 52
pityriasis versicolor, 46, 53
placental abruption, 125, 141
placenta praevia, 126–127, 142
plantar fasciitis, 165–166, 181
pleural effusion, 229, 241
pleural empyema, 229, 241
pneumatosis intestinalis, 10, 26
Pneumocystis jirovecii pneumonia (PJP), 243
pneumomediastinum, 231, 242
pneumonia
    community acquired, 233, 243
    lobar, 220, 238
    Pneumocystis jirovecii, 243
pneumonitis, hypersensitivity, 227, 240
pneumoperitoneum, 27
pneumothorax, 187–188, 203, 219, 229, 237, 241
    catamenial, 225, 240
    chylothorax, 224, 239
    primary spontaneous, 225, 240
    secondary spontaneous, 225, 239
    tension, 224, 239
Poikiloderma of Civatte, 46, 53
polycystic kidney disease, 196, 206
polycystic ovarian syndrome (PCOS), 109, 114, 124,
    135, 137, 140–141
polymorphous light eruption, 45, 53
polymyalgia rheumatica, 173, 177, 184, 186
pompholyx, 51
popcorn workers lung, 240
popliteal synovial cyst, 185
porphyria cutanea tarda, 34, 49
portal hypertension, 30
posterior cruciate ligament tear, 175, 186
posterior interosseus nerve syndrome, 164, 180
posterior shoulder dislocation, 176, 186
posterior vitreous detachment, 98, 107
post-nasal drip, 236
postpartum haemorrhage, 126, 142
post-thrombotic syndrome, 159, 178
post-traumatic stress disorder (PTSD), 60, 76
poxvirus, 30

pre-eclampsia, 87, 102, 125, 141
pregnancy, 108–109, 135
    ectopic, 126, 128, 142
    mask of, 54
pregnancy complications, 119–120, 139–140
premature ovarian failure, 123, 140
premenstrual dysphoric disorder, 57, 75
prepatellar bursitis, 174, 185
pre-prostatic and post-prostatic massage test
    (PPMT), 157
preterm premature rupture of membranes (PPROM),
    125, 141
primary biliary cirrhosis, 15, 28
primary ciliary dyskinesia, 117, 138
primary hyperaldosteronism, 195, 206
primary open angle glaucoma, 98, 107
primary ovarian insufficiency, 108, 135
primary sclerosing cholangitis, 15–16, 28
primary spontaneous pneumothorax, 225, 240
proctalgia fugax, 18, 29
prolactinoma, 109, 135
prostate cancer, 152–153, 157
prostatic hyperplasia, 151, 156
proximal interphalangeal (PIP) joints, 170, 183
pseudogout, 167, 182
pseudomembranous colitis, 4, 23
Pseudomonas aeruginosa, 140, 244
psittacosis, 226, 232, 240, 244
psoriasis, 37, 50, 120, 139
psoriatic arthritis, 169, 183
psychogenic non-epileptic seizures (PNES), 86, 102
pulmonary aspergillosis, 219, 237
pulmonary edema, acute, 223–224, 230, 239, 242
pulmonary embolism, 187, 190, 194, 203, 204, 206,
    222, 231, 238, 243
pulmonary regurgitation, 197, 207
pulmonary sequestration, 218, 237
pyloric stenosis, 9, 25, 26
pyoderma gangrenosum, 42, 52
pyogenic granuloma, 45, 53

R

radial tunnel syndrome, 164, 181
Ram's horn sign, 12, 27
Raynaud's phenomenon, 137, 182, 183
reactive arthritis, 185
rectal bleeding, 2
rectal prolapse, 18, 30
rectal varices, 19, 30
recurrent miscarriage, 120, 139
Reiter's syndrome, 175, 185
REM sleep behaviour disorder, 58, 75
renal artery stenosis, 195, 206
renal calculus, 134, 145, 153, 157, 161, 179
renal cell carcinoma, 151, 156

respiratory acidosis, 211–212, 234
respiratory alkalosis, 211–212, 234
respiratory diseases, 219–223, 237–239
respiratory microbiology, 243–244
respiratory syncytial virus (RSV), 236
restless leg syndrome, 59, 76
restrictive cardiomyopathy, 202, 210
retinal detachment, 99, 107
retinitis pigmentosa, 98, 107
retractile testicle, 149, 155
retropharyngeal abscess, 217, 236
rheumatic fever, 33, 48
rheumatoid arthritis, 171, 183
rhinitis medicamentosa, 214, 235
rhinosinusitis, acute, 88, 103, 215, 236
right bundle branch block, 192, 205
right coronary artery, 189, 204
ringworm, of scalp, 49
rodent ulcer, 52
roseola infantum, 33, 48
round atelectasis, 230, 242
runner's knee, 185
ruptured Baker's cyst, 174, 185
ruptured ectopic pregnancy, 132, 144
ruptured ovarian cyst, 132, 144

S

sabre-sheath trachea, 231, 242
sandblasting, 238, 240
saphena varix, 17, 29
sarcoidosis, 219, 237
scaphoid fracture, 170, 183
scarlet fever, 32, 48, 232, 243
Scheuermann's disease, 162, 179
schizoaffective disorder – bipolar type, 56, 75
schizoid personality disorder, 69, 80
schizophrenia, 55, 75
schizophreniform disorder, 56, 75
schizotypal personality disorder, 69, 80
Schwartz sign, 92, 104
scleroderma, 169, 182
scrotal abscess, 149, 155
scrotal calcinosis, 149, 155
scrotal disorders, see testicular and scrotal disorders
seborrheic dermatitis, 40, 51
seborrheic keratosis, 47, 54
secondary spontaneous pneumothorax, 225, 239
second-degree heart block – Mobitz type 2,
    192–193, 205
seizures, 85–88, 102–103, 191, 204
seminoma, 149, 155
separation anxiety disorder, 60, 76
septic arthritis, 175, 186
serotonin syndrome, 95, 106
Sever's disease, 167, 181

sexual health disorders of women, *see* female sexual
   health disorders
sexually transmitted infection, 129–130, 142–143
sexual masochism disorder, 66, 79
sexual sadism disorder, 67–68, 80
Shafer's sign, 107
shin splints, 160, 178
short gut syndrome, 4, 23
shoulder dislocation, posterior, 176, 186
shoulder dystocia, 126, 141
shoulder pain, *see* neck and shoulder pain
sialolithiasis, 88, 103
sigmoid volvulus, 10, 27
signet ring sign, 230, 242
sildenafil, 104
silicosis, 220, 227, 238, 240
simple partial seizure, 86, 102
skin infections, 32–33, 48
skin infections, in children, 32–34, 48
skin lesions, 44–45, 52–53
skin reactions, 34–35, 48–49
sleep disturbances, 58–59, 75–76
sleep terror, 58, 76
slipped capital femoral epiphysis, 173, 184
slipping rib syndrome, 188, 203
small bowel haematoma, 27
small bowel obstruction, 1–2, 22, 26
small cell lung carcinoma, 228, 241
small intestinal bacterial overgrowth
   (SIBO), 4, 23
snowman sign, 231, 242
social anxiety disorder, 60, 76
solar lentigo, 45, 53
solitary rectal ulcer syndrome, 19, 30
somnambulism, 59, 76
spermatocele, 149, 154
spinal abscess, 162, 179
spinal canal stenosis, 161, 179
spinal compression fracture, 162, 179
split pleura sign, 229, 241
spontaneous pneumothorax
   catamenial pneumothorax, 225, 240
   primary, 225, 240
   secondary, 225, 239
squamous cell carcinoma in situ, 44, 53
stack of coins sign, 12, 27
staphylococcal scalded skin syndrome, 34, 48
Staphylococcus aureus, 243
status migrainosus, 91, 104
Stevens-Johnson syndrome, 35, 49
Streptococcus pneumoniae, 243
Streptococcus pyogenes, 243
stress fracture, 168, 182
string of pearls sign, 11, 26
structural heart diseases, 200–202, 209–210
subarachnoid haemorrhage, 91, 104

substance related and addictive disorders, 70–72,
   80–81
subungual hematoma, 37, 50
superficial thrombophlebitis, 158, 178
supraspinatus tendon rupture, 177, 186
supraventricular tachycardia (SVT), 194, 205
surfer's ear, 105
sweet's syndrome, 42, 52
swimmer's ear, 235
syphilis, 130, 143
systemic lupus erythematosus (SLE), 169, 183

T

tacchycardia, 3
talon noir, 166–167, 181
target sign, 12, 27
tarsal tunnel syndrome, 167, 182
telltale triangle sign, 12, 27
telogen effluvium, 36, 49
temporal arteritis, 88–89, 103
temporomandibular joint dysfunction, 89, 103
tennis elbow, 180
tension headache, 89–90, 103
tension pneumothorax, 224, 239
teratoma, 151, 156
testicles, 138
testicular and scrotal disorders, 148–151, 154–156
testicular torsion, 149, 155
testis, gumma of, 148, 155
Tetralogy of Fallot, 202, 210, 230, 242
third-degree heart block, 194, 205
Thompson test, 178
threatened miscarriage, 119, 139
"thunderclap" headache, 104
tibialis posterior rupture, 160, 178
tinea capitis, 36, 49
tinea cruris, 149, 155
tinea nigra, 46, 54
tonic-clonic seizure, 88, 103
tonometry, 98
tonsillitis, 217, 237
torsion of hydatid of Morgagni, 149, 155
torticollis, 177, 186
total anomalous pulmonary venous return, 231, 242
Tourette syndrome, 95, 106
toxic megacolon, 3, 22
toxic pustuloderma, 49
Tracheo-Esophageal fistula, 215, 236
transient hip synovitis, 173, 184
transient ischaemic attack (TIA), 107
transposition of great arteries, 201, 209, 230, 242
transvestic disorder with fetishism, 67, 79
Treponema pallidum, 143
Trethowan's sign, 184
triangular cord sign, 31

trichilemmal cyst, 52
trichomoniasis, 129, 143
trichoscopy, 36
trichotillomania, 36, 49
tricuspid regurgitation, 197, 207
tricuspid stenosis, 198, 207
trigeminal nerve, 84, 101
trigeminal neuralgia, 88, 103
triptans, 104
Trisomy 21, 143
trochanteric bursitis, 172, 184
trochlear nerve, 83, 101
tuberculosis, 222, 238
tuberous sclerosis, 46, 53
Turner's syndrome, 108, 131, 135, 144
Turtle sign, 141
two-glass test, 157

U

ulcerative colitis, 4, 23, 27
ulcers, 8, 24–25
umbilical hernia, 16, 28
upper airway cough syndrome, 215, 236
urologic diseases, 151–153, 156–157
uroporphyrinogen decarboxylase (UROD), 48
uterine bleeding, dysfunctional, 115, 138
uterine fibroid, 114, 123, 137, 140
uterine polyp, 115, 137

V

valgus extension overload syndrome, 163, 180
varicella zoster virus, 48
varicoceles, 116, 117, 138, 150, 155–156
vascular dementia, 64, 78
vasovagal syncope, 191, 204

ventricular septal defect, 200, 209
vesicular hand dermatitis, 51
vestibular migraine, 84, 101
vestibular neuritis, 85, 101
vestibular schwannoma, 93, 105
viral esophagitis, 5, 23
viral infections, 203
vision loss, 98–99, 107
vitiligo, 47, 54
voice box, 237
vomiting, 9
Von Willebrand disease, 115, 137
voyeuristic disorder, 67, 79
vulvovaginal candidiasis, 122, 140
vulvovaginal disorders, 120–122, 139–140

W

Wartenberg's sign, 164, 180
water bottle sign, 230, 242
water-hammer pulse, 207
Wegener's granulomatosis, 213, 235, 239
Wernicke's encephalopathy, 64, 78
West syndrome, 86, 102
Williams syndrome, 130–131, 143
Willis–Ekbom disease, 76
Wilm's tumor, 9, 25, 153, 157
Wolff–Parkinson–White syndrome, 192, 205
women, sexual health disorders of, *see* female sexual
    health disorders
wrist disorders, *see* hand and wrist disorders
wry neck, 186

Y

yellow nail syndrome, 39, 51
Young's syndrome, 117, 138

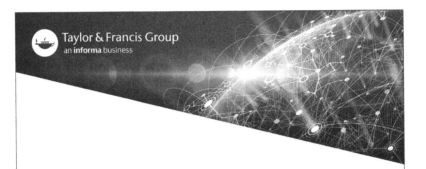

Printed in the United States
by Baker & Taylor Publisher Services